DID
YOUR
DOCTOR
TELL
YOU
?

PROFESSOR WILLEM SERFONTEIN

DID YOUR DOCTOR TELL YOU

?

MEDICAL MISCONCEPTIONS EXPOSED

Struik Publishers (a division of New Holland Publishing (South Africa) (Pty) Ltd)
New Holland Publishing is a member of Johnnic Communications Ltd

Cornelis Struik House, 80 McKenzie Street, Cape Town 8001, South Africa
86 Edgware Road, London, W2 2EA, United Kingdom
14 Aquatic Drive, Frenchs Forest, NSW 2086, Australia
218 Lake Road, Northcote, Auckland, New Zealand

www.struik.co.za

ISBN 1 86872 965 6

First published in 2004
10 9 8 7 6 5 4 3 2 1

Publishing manager: Linda de Villiers
Editors: Gail Jennings and Samantha Fick
Designer: Petal Palmer
DTP: Janine Cloete
Indexer: Cora Ovens

Reproduction: Hirt & Carter Cape (Pty) Ltd
Printing and binding: Paarl Print, Oosterland Street, Paarl, South Africa

Log onto our photographic website **www.imagesofafrica.co.za** for an African experience

www.imagesofafrica.co.za

IMAGES OF AFRICA
PHOTO LIBRARY

The views expressed in this book are those of the author and the publishers accept no responsibility for any action the reader may take as a result.

CONTENTS

DISCLAIMER   6

INTRODUCTION   7

CORONARY ARTERY DISEASE – IS CHOLESTEROL THE CULPRIT?   11

OSTEOPOROSIS – THE CALCIUM BANDWAGON   39

HRT ALERT   53

HIDDEN ANAEMIA AND EXCESSIVE IRON SUPPLEMENTATION   69

HIV/AIDS: ANOTHER PERSPECTIVE   79

CHEMOTHERAPY – OR NOT   103

LIFE-GIVING BACTERIA   123

MYTHS ABOUT MILK   131

THE MASS APPEAL OF MARGARINE   141

SOURCES OF NUTRIENTS   149

REFERENCES   151

INDEX   161

DISCLAIMER

This book provides information about nutrition and lifestyle as a way to help prevent and treat many of the most common chronic diseases that are on the increase today.

The information given is intended to serve as a guideline only and offers general recommendations. It should not be seen as prescriptive, nor is it the intention that the information be viewed as medical advice or advocating any substitution of medical prescriptions or diagnosis. It is intended to help you make informed decisions, and offer points of view, opinions and information other than those your health-care provider might have given you.

In all cases of serious illness, you should first consult a doctor or health-care provider you trust, and who has kept him- or herself up to date with objective medical and health trends and information.

Before you embark on any diet, supplementation programme or lifestyle change, or before you change any medication or treatment regime, it is advisable to discuss the matter with a practitioner who specialises in that particular field of health care.

The advice contained in this book is not intended as specific treatment. The author and the publisher do not accept any responsibility in this regard, nor do they guarantee that the use of the supplements or treatment regimes discussed are safe or effective in all cases.

INTRODUCTION

It's not surprising that everyone has an opinion about matters of health. After all, it is about life or death! And it's also not surprising that people have always looked up to those members of society – healers, midwives, doctors and medicine-makers – they believe are wise enough to be able to keep them healthy, and cure them when they're not.

Yet when it comes to health and wellbeing, wisdom is not cast in stone. What was regarded as a 'cure' a few hundred years ago, or even a few years ago, might later be discovered to be dangerous, harmful or simply ineffective. The problem is that ordinary people – those of us who seek medical help – don't always know about new developments in health and healing, and the sad truth is that our health-care practitioners don't always know, either.

Think about diseases such as coronary artery disease, osteoporosis, anaemia and cancer. We all 'know' the usual treatments and prevention measures: a low-cholesterol diet (with plenty of margarine and little animal fat), a diet high in calcium (plenty of milk and cheese), iron supplements and chemotherapy... Or do we?

This book takes time to investigate common wisdom and medical teachings about cholesterol, osteoporosis, hormone replacement therapy, HIV and AIDS, chemotherapy and anaemia, and offers second thoughts about the 'magic bullets' offered by the medical scientists and pharmaceutical industry.

There's plenty of evidence, as you will read in the pages that follow, to show that the medical and pharmaceutical industries don't always have our best interests at heart. You'll also read that the medical research industry has in some instances known for years (even decades) about dangers and alternatives to their proposed treatments, but have kept this information from you.

How is it possible that we have been betrayed by the very community that says it has committed itself to our wellbeing? How is it possible for medical scientists to ignore clear evidence that is contrary to so much of what they advocate and prescribe?

It is difficult to understand, but I suggest that personal pride in defending past attitudes, and especially the way in which medical opinion is shaped, may be involved. Medical opinion is shaped and formed by what the so-called 'opinion-makers' say. These are mostly esteemed elderly members of the profession who have long ago taken a certain stand on a particular issue and now feel compelled to defend that position in order not to lose face.

It is not difficult to find striking historical examples of this phenomenon.

THE SOILED FROCK SYNDROME

During the 1860s, bacteria and other disease-causing micro-organisms had not yet been discovered; indeed only a few microscopes existed in Europe. When French microbiologist Louis Pasteur therefore suggested that these micro-organisms not only do exist but that they are often the cause of many diseases, including infections, he was met with violent medical opposition and ridiculed for his new ideas. Since he was not a medical doctor but a scientist, he was accused of meddling in things about which he knew nothing!

At the same time a Viennese gynaecologist, Dr Semmelweiss, entered the picture. He met a similar barrage of criticism when he suggested that the extremely high mortality risk (20%) associated with child delivery as well as surgery (59%) could be drastically reduced by the simple matter of observing aseptic conditions during surgery and child delivery. He was ridiculed by his medical colleagues in Vienna to the extent that he was later barred from practising medicine. He fled to Paris, where a similar reception awaited him. He died in 1865, with no friends or money.

Both these pioneers were able to support their claims with evidence that was there for everyone to see. In the case of Dr Semmelweiss, he showed in clinical studies that the high mortality associated with childbirth could be reduced from nearly 20% to a mere 1% by washing hands and instruments during childbirth and surgery. In the case of Pasteur, the existence of micro-organisms could be demonstrated under the microscope (he owned one of the few in Europe).

These convincing experiments did nothing to convince the medical profession... but time would tell.

During the mid-1800s, doctors wore frock coats as 'badges' indicating their profession. These frock coats were often soiled with caked and dried blood, and surgeons would even keep in their coat lapels the hooks used to close wounds!

The turning point in what became known as the revolutionary 'germ theory of disease' came in 1881. Pasteur, using his theory about bacteria and their role in disease, prepared a vaccine against anthrax and demonstrated in a spectacular manner to the press and the whole world that he could protect sheep against anthrax by means of vaccination. The news spread like wildfire all over Europe, and overnight doctors cleaned up and discarded their blood-caked frocks and adopted aseptic procedures in child delivery and surgery.

All of a sudden Pasteur was a hero, and his vociferous medical critics disappeared.

It is remarkable that in spite of the rapid reaction in Europe, it took many years before doctors in America changed their views and practices, demonstrating how long it takes for new scientific discoveries to penetrate into general clinical practice (especially if established medical perceptions are supported by big industry!).

I predict that the 'refined polyunsaturated oil vs margarine saga' (see chapters one and nine) in relation to heart disease will one day be positioned next to the blood-caked frock episode in medical history.

More controversy awaits you as you read these pages... but it's not all controversy. These pages are committed to helping you make informed choices about the quality of your life.

CHAPTER ONE

CORONARY ARTERY DISEASE - IS CHOLESTEROL THE CULPRIT?

Coronary artery disease has defied the best attempts of the medical profession over the past 80 years. Known as CAD, this is a chronic disease of the vascular system that, despite research worth billions of dollars, remains the principal killer of human beings all over the world. And the billion dollar question is this: we know that CAD is a cause of heart attacks, but what is the cause of CAD? There is no doubt that cholesterol plays a role, but what is that role?

With CAD, plaque develops in the walls of the veins as a result of the accumulation of deposits (including cholesterol). Cholesterol is a fatty substance produced in the liver, and it plays an essential role in many life processes, including the biosynthesis of steroidal hormones.

When cholesterol levels are excessively high, a condition known as 'hyper-cholesterolaemia', it may cause deposits in the blood vessel wall, contributing to the formation of plaque. When the arteries become so narrow that the functioning of the heart muscle is compromised, or when a blood clot forms in these narrowed arteries, the result is a heart attack.

Between 1920 and 1960, CAD underwent a period of rapid increase, followed by a period of decline (1960–1990) in some countries such as the USA and Australia. But there is no indication that medical intervention had any influence on this decline!

This is largely because, as we shall see, the standard medical approach to prevent and treat the disease is seriously flawed. This treatment, which involves drug-induced lowering of cholesterol at all costs, disregards crucial facts about the disease.

A BRIEF HISTORY OF CAD SINCE 1900

Although the disease was described in medical texts before 1900, its incidence (the number of new cases) was extremely low during the first quarter of the 20th century, and was virtually unknown before 1926[16].

The occurrence of and death rate due to CAD in London hospitals between 1868 and 1980 was carefully studied and documented in 1980 by Dr R Finlayson from available hospital records[17]. He expressed his results as a ratio of the disease death rates per population sample, and this is what he found:

PERIOD OF TIME	CAD DEATH RATE RATIO
1869/1900	1
1900/1910	10
1900/1980	80

These figures show that the incidence of the disease was extremely low between 1869 and 1900, and remained virtually constant during this time interval. The figures also show that the death rate due to CAD had risen to such an extent by 1910 that the ratio (compared to 1900) was now 10, showing a 10-fold increase during this short period. In spite of this increase, the incidence of the disease compared to other diseases remained low; in 1926 it was still considered 'rare'[1].

After 1926 there was rapid escalation of the disease, because by 1980 the death rate ratio had risen to 80, showing that 80 times more people died of CAD in that year compared to 1900.

These observations were confirmed by a separate and independent study in Yorkshire by a Dr A Mackinnon[18]. This study was conducted in a constant rural population of 22 000, and confirmed both the 10-fold increase during 1900–1910 and the 80-fold increase between 1900 and 1980.

Both authors concluded that the 10-fold increase was due to the fact that mass-produced cigarettes had appeared on the market, and that 80% of men were smoking them. Both authors did not comment on the fact that a much larger increase in death rate due to CAD occurred after 1910 and presumably after 1926, since it was reported in that year that CAD was still a rare disease.

The relevance of cigarette smoking remains undisputed, but the above figures suggest that while it is indeed an important cause of our present-day problems, it is not the main cause.

More likely, the most important causes of CAD occurred after 1926, as a result of industrialisation and urbanisation, and its resulting lifestyle changes and increased consumption of refined carbohydrates.

THE IMPACT OF REFINED FLOUR

Before 1900, most bread was made of wholegrain wheat, which contained a variety of minerals and vitamins as well as small but vital quantities of essential fatty acids and antioxidant tocopherols. Tocopherols are the different forms of vitamin E that occur in nature, and are powerful antioxidants because of their ability to react and remove the dangerous free radicals in the body that may result from inhaled industrial toxins.

Around 1900, roller mills were introduced in Europe and the USA, which greatly facilitated the milling of wheat. The immediate result was that wheat could be ground to a much finer flour, and this refinement could be carried out on a massive industrial scale. Finely ground flour has a much higher glycaemic index[19] than the coarser variety, which means that blood sugar levels rise much more sharply after eating refined flour than unrefined flour.

This is because milling greatly reduces the particle size in wheat, and particle size is the factor in the glycaemic index. This in turn has a big influence on insulin resistance and therefore on CAD. Briefly, insulin resistance refers to a situation where more and more insulin is required to keep the glucose at an even level in the blood. When insulin levels are high (reflecting insulin resistance), blood sugar levels tend to be high, and this has important health consequences, including an increased risk of CAD and diabetes.

However, it is not only particle size that changes during the process of food refinement; up to 90% of the vital vitamins and minerals are also removed. Many of these are of specific importance in relation to the problem of CAD, especially the protective antioxidant tocopherols that are removed in the bran fraction.

In addition, the newly refined wheat flour is treated with bleaching agents such as chlorine dioxide (a powerful oxidising agent) in order to improve its appearance. These bleaching agents further destroy whatever small quantities of antioxidants and other vital nutrients remains in the refined flour.

THE FACTS ABOUT CAD

➤ CAD is still the leading cause of death in Europe and the USA (between a third and a quarter of all deaths), despite 50 years of medical advice and many millions spent on drugs and research.

➤ The USA is the only country in which there has been a major decline in CAD (40%), and it is also the only country in which there has been a major increase in vitamin C consumption (300%). The relevance of vitamin C is that mammals that manufacture their own vitamin C (in their liver) do not develop the same type of cardiovascular lesions as humans do (humans do not make vitamin C). (See the vitamin C theory of heart disease, page 31.)

➤ Despite the medical profession's heavy emphasis on cholesterol levels, more than 60% of heart patients do not have raised blood cholesterol levels[6].

➤ At least 30 randomised intervention clinical trials (the most accurate form of study) investigating different means of lowering cholesterol have been completed during the last 30 years in the developed world, at a cost exceeding $1 000 million[19]. Each has investigated the efficacy of cholesterol lowering as a tool to control CAD.

➤ It is rare for a vein to develop plaques. Instead, plaques are often localised in arteries close to the heart, where arterial pressure is maximal, and where damage to collagen and elastin structures in the arteries may reasonably be expected to be greatest. Vitamin C is a critical factor in the repair and maintenance of such structures.

➤ Elevated cholesterol levels (reflecting elevated LDL – 'bad' cholesterol levels) have been shown in many studies to be strongly associated with CAD, but most of these studies were done before the distinction between LDL and Lipoprotein a (Lpa) had been defined. (Lpa is a related lipid made in the body from LDL.) Therefore what was described in these studies as 'LDL' was actually LDL+Lpa. Lpa is a stronger indicator of risk than LDL[11].

➤ Approximately 50% of all people below the age of 50 who die from CAD do not have any of the known risk factors, including abnormal cholesterol values[19]. At least two population studies have shown that while lowering cholesterol levels may lead to reduction in CAD mortality, this reduction is largely offset by a rise in cancer deaths.

WHAT CAUSES CAD?

A problem with this question is the abundance of theories about the cause of CAD. It is thus extremely difficult for anyone, scientists included, to decide on which one.

There is the cholesterol theory (that high blood cholesterol levels cause the disease), the fat theory (that too much saturated fat and too little polyunsaturated fats are the cause of cholesterol), and the important homocysteine theory (that rising homocysteine levels in the blood, perhaps due to vitamin deficiencies, are the cause).

There's also the oxidised cholesterol theory (which states that cholesterol becomes dangerous only once it is oxidised); the free radical heavy metal theory (that excessive free radical activity arising from low levels of antioxidants and increased levels of certain micro-minerals, including iron, are the cause); and even a microbe theory (that vascular infections by certain 'stealth organisms' are the cause).

With so many possibilities, it is extremely unlikely that any one measure, such as the lowering of blood cholesterol levels, will deliver a solution to the problem.

THE 'FAT THEORY' OF CAD

The 'fat theory' indicates that a high dietary fat intake causes blood cholesterol levels to rise – high cholesterol is the result of a high fat intake. This then causes accumulation of cholesterol in the artery walls, which leads to heart attacks. The cholesterol theory also identifies cholesterol as the culprit when it comes to heart attacks, but notes that this cholesterol could have been raised as a result of a genetic predisposition or a high intake of refined sugars, for example.

There is a substantial body of evidence that contradicts these theories, though. Around 1900, when the incidence of CAD was extremely low, fats in the diet consisted mainly of lard and butter, which according to present-day medical teachings are the principal causes of CAD. Margarine as we know it today, and refined vegetable fats such as commercial sunflower oil, did not yet exist. What little margarine was available before 1910 was produced from tallow and coconut oil (both predominantly saturated fats).

Today's products are produced by means of the catalytic hydrogenation of refined vegetable oils, from which the protective antioxidant tocopherols had been removed. These new margarines became popular during the period 1910 to 1920, precisely when there was a rapid rise in the incidence of CAD.

During the 1940s, polyunsaturated vegetable oils and margarine attracted much media and medical attention when it was found that they had a mild cholesterol-lowering effect in human experiments. Believing cholesterol to be the principal cause of CAD, the medical profession therefore decided that margarine and the vegetable oils from which it was made were 'good', and that saturated fats such as lard and butter were 'bad'.

Unfortunately, that is still their teaching today, disregarding the findings of Finlayson and Mackinnon as well as those of more recent studies, which show that communities such as the Masai in East Africa consume large quantities of saturated fats yet have a very low incidence of CAD.

THE ANTIOXIDANT CONNECTION

In the 1970s Prof Anderson of the University of Toronto, Canada, provided evidence that polyunsaturated maize oil from which the antioxidants had been removed was damaging to the hearts of experimental animals[20]. He linked this observation to the enormous increase in death rates due to CAD, as the intake of polyunsaturated oil increased and as the refinement of bread became standard practice.

He cites supporting evidence from several sources. The first is the recorded incidence of CAD in Italy during the period 1919 to 1946. In 1919 the refinement and bleaching of flour was banned in Italy, in order to reduce the country's dependence on imported wheat. The ban was maintained until 1946, during which time there was no increase in CAD deaths or incidence in Italy. In the other European countries and in the USA, deaths due to CAD increased by more than 200% during this period (we do not have figures for incidence rates).

Other observational studies supported the conclusions drawn from the Italian experience. One study, concluded in 1992, compared the incidence of CAD deaths in the south of France with that in Scotland. The two study populations were similar in many respects and even the serum cholesterol values were the same in the two populations (approximately 6,0 mmol/l). Yet the death rate due to CAD was five times higher in Scotland than in France[21]. This difference was attributed to the high consumption of wine in France. The average adult in the south of France consumes 500 ml of red wine every day, which contains 100 mg of flavonoid antioxidants.

The antioxidant (and specifically the bioflavonoid antioxidant) connection was further supported by observations made in the Zutphen cohort (follow-up) study in the 1980s in the Netherlands. Here again the consumption of a bioflavonoid (quercitin) was related to the incidence of CAD mortality. It was found that men who consumed (from the diet) less than 10 mg per day of quercitin had a 200% increase in the CAD death rate, compared to those who consumed more than 30 mg. The main dietary sources of quercitin were onions, apples and black tea. Increased quercitin in the diet was also found to be associated with a reduced mortality rate from all causes.

These and other studies have established beyond doubt the connection between antioxidant intake and the CAD mortality rate, but the precise mechanisms involved remained to be elucidated.

NOT ALL 'GOOD' FATS ARE GOOD

Recent studies have linked the intake of refined polyunsaturated fatty acids (such as refined plant oils and margarine) and heart disease. That's because polyunsaturated fatty acids (PUFAs), by virtue of their chemical structure, are highly susceptible to attack by oxygen in the air. In reacting with oxygen, these PUFAs are easily converted into what's known as hydroperoxides, which are highly reactive free radicals. These free radicals are capable of attacking and destroying the membranes in many critical sites in the body, including brain cells and artery walls. Free radical attack on arterial walls is generally assumed to contribute significantly to the process of atherosclerosis.

Atherosclerosis, or the hardening of the arteries, refers to the appearance of plaque in the vascular walls. Adequate levels of antioxidants not only prevent the formation of hydroperoxides but also protect against tissue damage that may be caused by these free radicals. Hydroperoxides are also highly damaging to the sensitive cells of the immune system, and are therefore strongly immunosuppressive.

Small quantities of certain PUFAS (omega-3 and omega-6) are essential for good health, and in order to prevent deficiencies, many people take supplements in the form of fish oil, evening primrose oil and flaxseed oil. However, the fatty acids in these supplements, especially those in flaxseed oil, are also susceptible to oxidation, with the same resulting harmful consequences that occur in refined plant oils. Such supplements should therefore always be taken in combination with adequate quantities of antioxidants such as vitamin E.

THE PRUDENT DIET

The Prudent Diet was developed in medical circles in the mid-1950s in response to the theory that raised cholesterol levels are the principal cause of CAD and therefore heart attacks. Focusing mainly on fat intake, this diet was based on several findings that showed that the PUFAs in the diet reduced cholesterol levels by about 10%.

Medical opinion therefore decided that the fat component of our diets should consist of at least two-thirds PUFAs, with the other third in the form of mainly saturated fats.

The Prudent Diet was introduced with great fanfare, proclaiming to be the solution to heart problems. Most doctors and medical opinion-makers of the time enthusiastically supported it. Thousands of patients were put on this diet, while large numbers of the public were advised to do likewise in order to avoid a heart attack.

I was one of the medical researchers who supported the programme at the time. However, not everyone did so. One exception was Dr Paul Dudley White, personal cardiologist to the USA's President Eisenhower. Dr White pointed out that he had been a practising cardiologist since 1921 and that during those years he had seen a dramatic increase in the incidence of CAD, including the last number of years during which the Prudent Diet had been introduced.

He saw his first case of CAD in 1931, and his colleagues travelled from afar to see this case of a new and rare cause of heart attack. He also pointed out that before the 1930s, when CAD was virtually absent from the population, the diet consisted largely of butter, lard and high cholesterol foods[15].

However, his lonely voice did not stem the growing flood of influential supporters of this Prudent Diet, especially since the pharmaceutical industry was now engaged enthusiastically in the development of cholesterol-lowering drugs. Further support for this diet came from the food industry, which was supplying the low-cost polyunsaturated oils for the manufacture of margarine – which had the effect of pricing butter out of the market.

The combined effect of widespread support by the medical profession as well as the co-operation of the pharmaceutical and food industries was that the PUFA intake in our diet increased by 300%, while lard virtually disappeared from food shelves, accompanied by a substantial reduction in butter sales.

This situation has persisted to the present day, with many doctors and even the Heart Foundation still telling the public that margarine and polyunsaturated oils are good.

It is important to note that all of this happened without direct clinical proof that the Prudent Diet was beneficial. Not too long afterwards, the first clinical trials were initiated, and below is a summary of Dr Wayne Martin's account of what happened.

The Joliffe Anticoronary Club Trial

The Joliffe Anticoronary Club Trial[26] was conducted by Dr Joliffe in New York in the 1960s. Dr Joliffe was seriously ill, in a wheelchair, with advanced diabetes and its complications (vascular lesions in the eyes and ulceration in one foot). He was convinced that the Prudent Diet would help him get over his health problems, so he recruited men, mostly teachers in colleges and universities, to join him in the active group on the Prudent Diet in this trial.

The controls were mostly wealthy businessmen living on the typical high-cholesterol and high-fat diet of the rich. In this diet, as opposed to the Prudent Diet, the fats were nearly all of the saturated type, thought to be the main cause of heart disease.

The selection of the active group and control groups from two dissimilar population groups made the trial flawed as a valid scientific instrument (to ensure lack of bias and error it is essential that the active group and the controls are as similar as possible). This selection bias created the impression that the trial had been designed to ensure an outcome in favour of the Prudent Diet. The trial ran for six years, and the results were published in the *Journal of the American Medical Association* in 1966. These showed that, as expected, average cholesterol values declined by 10%.

This result was hailed as a great success by the medical and the lay press, and again it was claimed that the Prudent Diet would prevent heart attacks, since it was inconceivable that lowering of cholesterol would not be accompanied by a reduction in risk.

The public was therefore not told that the number of coronary deaths was exactly the opposite of what was expected – eight people died in the Prudent Diet group and none in the control group. This was followed by the death of Dr Joliffe himself.

The unexpected mortality figures were considered to be due to chance, since the numbers involved in the trial were relatively small. Dr Joliffe's death was attributed to his diabetic condition.

The reaction of the medical profession was to suggest that the trial should then be immediately followed by a follow-on trial involving a million men. The new trial was to be called the National Diet Heart Study, and it was to be run by the National Heart Institute with funding from the US Government. Dr Irvine Page of the Cleveland Clinic was in charge of the new study.

Dr Martin tells of discussions he had with Dr Page[15], a heart attack survivor himself. Dr Page was confident of the success of the proposed study, and was convinced that the diet would prevent him from having another heart attack.

The trial was elaborately planned. Food warehouses were set up in five cities where trial participants could get free food with the correct composition and polyunsaturated fatty acid content (polyunsaturated doughnuts, and meat from which every trace of fat had been trimmed away). Control subjects received a normal diet.

Before embarking on the full trial, it was wisely decided to run a pretrial involving only 2 000 men, aged 45 to 54, and divided into two equal randomised groups. (In this context, randomised does not mean 'random', but means instead that each person has an equal chance of being selected for either group, thus minimising bias and ensuring an equal spread of possible confounding factors.)

The trial was run over a six-year period, the results of which were published in the journal Circulation[27]. As expected, there was a lowering of cholesterol in the Prudent Diet group from 6,5 to 5,85 mmol/l and this, in turn, prompted one group of cardiologists to proclaim the pretrial a success and insist on the immediate instigation of the main trial.

However, many other cardiologists were hesitant, since no clinical advantage of the Prudent Diet over controls could be demonstrated, as the same number of participants in both groups had died during the trial. The number of non-fatal heart attacks in the two groups was also the same.

As a result of this, the grandiose projected trial was quietly abandoned, 'for reasons of cost'. The public and the scientific community were not advised that the trial had failed to demonstrate a clinical advantage associated with the Prudent Diet.

We still hear medical doctors, dieticians and even the Heart Foundation talking about the benefits of margarine and polyunsaturated oils to prevent heart attacks.

This in spite of these and many other similar studies which show that not only do they not have any clinical advantages, but may in fact increase the risk[28]. They certainly do not increase the survival rate[19].

Population studies

The failure of these two direct clinical trials to demonstrate any clinical advantage of the Prudent Diet was perceived to be due to unexplained shortcomings in the study designs. There have been no other clinical trials investigating this diet.

But such was the fervour and enthusiasm of some cardiologists for the Prudent Diet that they now sought other avenues to prove its value after all. The next avenue to investigate was the incidence of CAD in different communities with different dietary habits. These dietary habits were such that they should yield information on the impact of polyunsaturated oils on the incidence of heart attack deaths.

The Boston-Ireland brothers study

The people in the Boston area in the United States were living on a diet close to the Prudent Diet, whereas Ireland at that time was a principally dairy nation, where the market for butter was protected by the restrictions on the importation of low-cost polyunsaturated oils and margarines. As a result of this, the average adult consumption of butter in Ireland was nearly 500 g per week, with virtually no vegetable oils or margarines.

This offered a good opportunity to compare the incidence of heart attacks in the two populations and to reach conclusions regarding the benefits or otherwise of the polyunsaturates[29]. Dr Stare, the organiser of the trial, succeeded in identifying families in Ireland in which one brother had immigrated to the Boston area while the other had remained in Ireland. It was expected to find that the Boston brothers had a lower incidence of heart attacks than their Irish brothers.

Exactly the opposite was found. The Boston brothers had a much higher incidence of heart attacks than their Irish brothers[20].

This was big news in the USA, and the cardiologists suggested that the result could be explained by the fact that the Irish brothers did much more walking, and that this had prevented the heart attacks in spite of the high intake of butter. While exercise could indeed have been a factor, the fact still had to be faced that a high-fat diet does not necessarily cause heart attacks!

The Roseto study

Roseto is a small town in Pennsylvania with a near 100% Italian population. It was known that the incidence of heart attacks is lower in Italy and also in Roseto than elsewhere. In addition, the incidence of CAD among the Italians in Roseto was much lower than that among their Pennsylvania Dutch neighbours.

The dietary habits in the two populations were radically different. The Italians were relatively prosperous and their diet consisted mainly of high-fat meatballs and a good deal of Italian cheese, with almost no polyunsaturates.

This offered a good opportunity to conduct a more detailed study of the incidence of heart attacks in the two populations and to draw conclusions regarding the value of the Prudent Diet, which was very similar to that followed by the neighbouring Dutch and the rest of the US population at that time.

Prof Wolf at the University of Oklahoma conducted such a study[30]. The results showed that the incidence of heart attacks in Roseto, with the high saturated fat diet, was one third lower than in the rest of the USA.

Again the result was surprising, and cardiologists suggested that the difference in heart attack incidence could be due to the fact that the Italians were 'members of a large family, which reduced the stresses of life'. Nevertheless, on a comparison of diet alone, ingestion of high-fat foods was once again shown to not necessarily result in a heart attack.

Indian population study

Dr Malhotra in India conducted a study of the incidence of heart attacks in two population groups in India with radically different dietary habits[31].

One group was in the north, where there was an extremely high consumption of butter in the form of ghee (clarified butter). Although members of this group also consumed some meat, the bulk of their diet consisted of wholegrain wheat. These people had a very low incidence of heart attacks.

The other group consisted of people in the south of the country where the diet, presumably because of economic considerations, was similar to the Prudent Diet. Here the principal dietary fat components were polyunsaturated fats in the form of peanut oil and the margarine made from it. They ate almost no saturated fats.

The results of the study showed that there were nearly 15 times more heart attacks among the Prudent Diet followers in the south than among those in the north.

Later it was reported that there was a vast increase in heart attacks in the north when the low-cost polyunsaturated vegetable oils and margarines had virtually priced ghee out of the market[32].

WHAT CAN WE CONCLUDE?

The collective evidence suggests that refined polyunsaturated oils and margarines not only are ineffective in preventing heart attacks, but in fact may cause them.

While these fats do lower cholesterol, this lowering does not have a large effect on the risk of heart attacks. And as the majority of heart patients do not have raised cholesterol values, it is wrong to treat everyone at risk for a heart attack with a cholesterol-lowering drug.

How is it possible that the 'fat theory' could prevail despite clear evidence to the contrary that has been collected since the 1960s? I suggest that personal pride may be involved. Medical opinion is shaped and formed by so-called 'opinion makers', who are mostly esteemed elderly members of the profession who have long ago taken a stand on a particular issue and feel compelled to defend that position in order not to lose face.

THE 'CHOLESTEROL THEORY' OF CAD

The cholesterol theory of CAD states that saturated animal fats in the diet cause blood cholesterol to rise, promoting the deposition of cholesterol in the artery walls. This then leads to the accumulation of plaque (the arterial deposits seen in the arteries of heart patients).

Few other theories – not even the polyunsaturated margarine saga – have inspired more heated debate and controversy in medical circles than the cholesterol theory. Today there is much evidence that suggests that saturated animal fats cause cholesterol levels to rise only if the intake of refined carbohydrates is also high (and, of course, the question still remains as to whether cholesterol is the culprit in CAD anyway)!

Currently the medical profession is solidly behind the cholesterol theory, and a statin drug to lower cholesterol levels is prescribed to virtually every heart patient, even when these levels are only slightly elevated.

The statins are a new class of drugs that are effective cholesterol-lowering agents, and several well-conducted clinical studies have been completed that show that these drugs effectively lower blood cholesterol values and may also have short-term advantages in terms of patient survival.

However, it needs to be asked whether cholesterol-lowering is in fact the most effective means of reducing heart risk. And if so, are the statins the most effective and safest drugs to use for cholesterol lowering?

There is little doubt that increased levels of blood cholesterol levels are associated with an increased risk of heart disease and stroke. This is confirmed by the results of many reputable studies[33]. However, these studies do not isolate a high cholesterol blood level as the only or even the principal cause of heart attacks in general.

While the association between an analytical total blood cholesterol level reading and heart risk is not in real dispute, the practical significance of this is very much in dispute. In particular, it is by no means certain that lowering of raised blood cholesterol levels artificially is beneficial in all age groups and under all circumstances. It is wrong, and possibly harmful, to prescribe a cholesterol-lowering drug to anyone with a moderately raised cholesterol level (especially in the aged) without first considering other possible causes, such as hormonal imbalances (see pages 30–31).

CHOLESTEROL FRACTIONS IN THE BLOOD

The total blood cholesterol reading reflects the sum total of different cholesterol fractions, including the LDL fraction (low-density lipoprotein, the so-called 'bad' cholesterol) and the HDL fraction (high-density lipoprotein, the 'good' cholesterol).

Many studies have shown that it may be more important to maintain high levels of the beneficial HDL than it is to suppress high levels of LDL[34]. This has clear implications for the risk evaluation of a particular total cholesterol reading. In addition, Lpa, a fatty, cholesterol-bearing lipoprotein that occurs naturally in the blood (and which is usually lumped together with LDL), and oxidised cholesterol are other important forms of cholesterol in the blood.

OXIDISED CHOLESTEROL

A number of scientists now believe that LDL itself is not dangerous; the real culprit is the oxidised LDL cholesterol formed in the blood from LDL when there is a deficiency of protective antioxidants such as vitamins C and E and coenzyme Q10[35].

Guarding against LDL cholesterol oxidation protects against atherosclerosis as well as heart attacks[36].

It is of particular interest to note that DHEA (dihydroepiandrosterone, the direct precursor of testosterone and the oestrogens) forms a part of the protective 'shield' in the LDL molecule (along with vitamin E) that protects it against oxidation. Vitamin E does not fully protect LDL against oxidation unless adequate levels of DHEA are present[38].

This may explain why some elderly people are particularly susceptible to atherosclerosis and the effects of LDL oxidation, since it is known that DHEA levels may be extremely low in such people. Population studies have shown that DHEA levels in the elderly decline to less than 20% of those in healthy young people.

Although oxidised LDL cholesterol is probably the real culprit, it is important to guard against the excessive accumulation of LDL cholesterol, as analytically no distinction is made between ordinary LDL and oxidised LDL. Elevated LDL is important in all patients, but especially in the elderly[37]. There appears to be a point in some people when the process of atherosclerosis accelerates, which may be related to the individual's DHEA, as noted above. If this happens, even slightly elevated LDL levels may be dangerous[39].

So although these findings cast doubt on the direct interpretation of a particular cholesterol reading, health conscious people should certainly not disregard the importance of cholesterol values. When these values are elevated (eg above 6,0 mmol/l), especially if you are under the age of 40, you should make every attempt to reduce these to more acceptable levels. How best to achieve this is the issue (see page 29).

On the other hand, the exaggerated importance attached to cholesterol in relation to heart risk is certainly wrong and misleading. There are many doctors who will put a patient with a cholesterol value of 5,4 mmol/l on a statin drug in order to reduce the value to below 5,0 mmol/l. This is not only unfounded, but may be harmful (see page 27).

With regard to stroke, high cholesterol levels definitely increase the risk of one type of stroke (the more common ischaemic type) but on the other hand, cholesterol values that are too low (eg below 4,0 mmol/l), may increase the risk for hemorrhagic stroke due to weakened vascular walls[40].

THE STATIN DRUGS

Over the last few decades many different cholesterol-lowering drugs have been developed in an attempt to stem the tide of heart attack deaths.

At least 30 different clinical studies at an estimated total cost exceeding $1 billion have been completed to test the hypothesis that such deaths can be lowered by reducing blood cholesterol levels by means of some of these drugs[41]. None of these studies have shown conclusively that cholesterol lowering has any real advantages for the patient in the long term, yet many yielded negative results even in the short term.

Trials such as the Lipid Research Clinics Coronary Prevention Trial (which cost $175 million) showed, in 1984, that in the short-term mortality due to a heart attack was reduced after drug-induced cholesterol lowering, but that overall mortality was the same in trial and control groups due to increased mortality associated with other causes, such as the increased cancer incidence following cholesterol lowering[42]. (Cholesterol is a key factor in the membrane structure of cells, and faulty membranes are associated with an increased cancer risk.)

Then in the 1980s the statins were introduced, so named because they are supposed to keep the cholesterol levels static, and today they are among the most frequently prescribed drug classes in the world. They are not only very effective at lowering cholesterol, but several clinical studies have shown that they also reduce CAD mortality, at least in the short term.

The most important of these statin intervention studies was the Scandinavian Simvastatin Survival Study[43]. The results, published in 1994, were in direct contrast to those obtained in a large number of other studies in many parts of the world.

The Simvastatin Study revealed that, not only were cholesterol levels significantly reduced – at least in those heart patients with elevated cholesterol levels – but also that the treatment was clinically beneficial in the short term (approximately five years).

The survival rate in the treated group after five years was more than 30% better than in the control group. Other studies, including one in healthy people with raised cholesterol levels, yielded similar results.

Collectively, these results finally confirmed to many medical doctors that the concept of cholesterol lowering is the way to go to prevent and treat heart disease; the use of statins in such patients has virtually become standard medical practice.

However, very few doctors have paused to consider the almost 30 other cholesterol-lowering studies, using different cholesterol-lowering methods, which have shown very little or no benefit in heart patients. Indeed, this has prompted the suggestion that the benefits associated with the statins might have little to do with their effects on cholesterol levels!

This suggestion has been confirmed after a study published in 2002[44], and researchers have begun to talk about the 'extra lipid' effects of the statins. This refers to the stabilising effect that the statins have on plaque deposits, thus preventing them from breaking up and causing heart attacks, and also perhaps because the statins have antioxidant properties.

The downside of the statins

It came as a shock to millions of doctors and patients alike when in 2002 the drug company Bayer announced that it was withdrawing its cholesterol-lowering drug cerevastatin ('Baycol') with immediate effect.

The reason was the increasing reports of side effects involving muscular weakness (rhabdomyolysis), especially when the statin was used with certain other cholesterol lowering measures. Rhabdomyolysis is a rare, potentially life-threatening condition, first manifested by muscle pain but which may progress to kidney failure and death. Approximately 53 deaths had been recorded by the time the drug was withdrawn.

Cerevastatin was one of five statin products on the South African market, and it does appear to be more toxic than the other statins. Nevertheless, the European Medicines Evaluation Agency (EMEA) decided in August 2001 that it was going to review the safety and status of all the other statins. The results of the review have not yet been published.

This came as a great disappointment to doctors, because they like the statins for the simple reason that they work, at least as far as the lowering of cholesterol and the short-term survival rates are concerned. Unfortunately, like all other drugs, these impressive short-term beneficial effects have serious long-term side effects; with statins this is particularly serious, since these drugs have to be used virtually indefinitely.

Also of concern is the way statin drugs lower the levels of coenzyme Q10, especially in the mitochondria (the structures inside cells where energy is generated from carbohydrate and fat fuel molecules). Q10 is one of the critical coenzymes required in the mitochondria for the production of energy. Reduced mitochondrial energy production (from free radical damage) is the hallmark of the cancer cell[45].

The key intermediate in the pathways that lead to the synthesis of both cholesterol and coenzyme Q10 is mevalonate and, as noted above, its synthesis is blocked by the statins. Many of the long-term side effects of the statins can be directly linked to this critical lowering (45–75%) of Q10 levels.

HIDDEN SIDE EFFECTS OF STATINS

➤ **Increased cancer risk: All statins have been shown to cause cancer in experimental animals[46], with reference to the connection between low mitochondrial Q10 levels and cancer. This does not mean that that the same risk exists in humans, but it does indicate possible risk.**

➤ Suppression of insulin and antioxidant levels: A 2001 Finnish study in men with high cholesterol levels found that treatment with simvastatin (Zocor) resulted in a reduction of cholesterol levels (20,8%), but insulin levels were increased by 13% and antioxidant levels (including Q10) declined by 22%. Glucose levels were not affected, suggesting a decrease in insulin sensitivity. The serious long-term effects of rising Insulin levels and decreased insulin sensitivity include increased diabetic tendencies, with all their accompanying side effects such as an increased risk of heart attacks.

➤ Weakening of the heart muscle with increased risk of cardiomyopathy (weakness to the extent that the heart pumping action is compromised): Q10 is critically important for energy production in the heart muscle, and the use of the statin class of drugs has been associated with an increased incidence of cardiomyopathy[47].

➤ Undesirable effects on the immune system: These side effects include the suppression of helper T-cells[48].

➤ Peripheral neuropathy: Nerve function may be affected by the statins, and typical symptoms are weakness and pain in hands and feet. The results of a Danish study published in 2002 show that users of statins were at least four times more likely to develop polyneuropathy than non-users.

➤ Statins increase levels of Lpa: this therefore increases cardiovascular risk[48].

Some of the other documented side effects of the statins include muscle damage, cramps, elevation of muscle enzymes, abnormal electromyograms, gastro-intestinal problems, dizziness, sleep problems, liver problems and sexual dysfunction[50]. They also may cause anxiety and depression, optic nerve degeneration and impair the growth of brain cells[51].

This formidable list of documented side effects has not yet attracted the attention of the medical profession, and only some are listed on the drug packaging.

The risk of developing any single one of these side effects is perhaps small, but taken together the total risk is not one that can be disregarded.

When should cholesterol levels be lowered?
Cholesterol is neither the only nor even the principal cause of heart attacks. However, when cholesterol is grossly elevated, for example due to a genetic defect (familial

hypercholesterolaemia) with blood levels of say above 7,0 mmol/l, then it does become a serious risk factor and it should be lowered, even with the use of drugs if necessary.

On the other hand, cholesterol is essential for life, and blood levels that are too low also constitute a risk factor for diseases such as stroke. When levels are raised as a result of other factors (such as diet and lifestyle), elevations of blood cholesterol are usually less severe (between 6,0 and 7,0 mmol/l), which is why these changes should always be the first option before drugs.

It is wrong to prescribe a drug to lower a blood cholesterol level of say 5,8 mmol/l.

Do the advantages of statins outweigh the disadvantages?

No real long-term advantages of the statins have been demonstrated, and although the collective disadvantages are difficult to quantify, they are always present in a subtle way. One of these is the risk of developing 'unexplained' cardiomyopathy after 10 years, in addition to the other problems for which statins are prescribed.

What are the alternatives?

The use of the statins is justified in the high-risk patient with substantially raised cholesterol levels (above 8,0 mmol/l) who doesn't respond to other risk reduction measures such as diet and lifestyle (increased exercise and reduced intake of refined foods).

In such cases the objective must be to phase out the drugs, or at least reduce dosage levels, while other less dangerous procedures are introduced. However, it is unfortunately true that, until recently, there have been no natural products that will lower cholesterol as effectively as drugs such as the statins. Vitamin B3 (niacin) and some of its derivatives could be considered, but they too have unpleasant side effects.

Fortunately a new natural product, Policosanol, has appeared on the market, and it appears to be as effective as, if not better than, the statins. It also offers additional advantages without any of the harmful side effects of the statins, and consists of a mixture of eight or nine long-chain alcohols obtained from the leaves of the sugar cane plant.

Policosanol has an unexpected number of beneficial effects for the heart patient, and a surprisingly large number of clinical studies (including comparative studies with some of the statin drugs) have already been completed. These studies show that Policosanol works better than the statins to lower blood cholesterol while at the same time raising levels of the 'good' cholesterol. It also lowers blood triglycerides and suppresses blood clotting[52].

It acts by blocking the synthesis of cholesterol but it achieves this by means of a mechanism that differs from that of the statins. It does not block HMG-CoA reductase like the statins, and therefore does not have the adverse effects that the statins have on Q10 levels (hence the absence of side effects).

Other direct beneficial clinical effects in the heart patient include a reduction of artery lesions that lead to atherosclerosis[53], and it also prevents the chronic inflammatory response associated with the oxidation of cholesterol[54]. Furthermore, it inhibits the formation of blood clots[55] and does not interfere with other heart drugs.

Why has the medical profession taken so little notice of Policosanol? Perhaps because it is a harmless natural product that cannot be patented and therefore does not enjoy the millions of dollars invested in the marketing of the statins to the medical profession.

Patients who are already on statin therapy should not make any drastic changes on their own, or even switch over to Policosanol without first consulting their doctor. It is best to talk to your doctor and then jointly decide on the most beneficial programme of action in your particular case.

THE 'HORMONE IMBALANCE' THEORY

In 2003 two American researchers, Drs SA Dzugan and RA Smith, published the results of a study conducted over five years (1997–2002) on 41 patients with raised cholesterol levels. This study may forever change our thinking about cholesterol and the way we treat elevated levels.

As opposed to conventional wisdom that raised blood cholesterol levels are due either to excessive production (in the liver) or excessive dietary intake, these researchers found that another cause of rising cholesterol levels are the age-related declining levels of hormones in the blood. In the elderly, these hormone imbalances may be the principal cause of raised cholesterol[230].

All steroid hormones are produced in the body from cholesterol, which is why cholesterol is known as the precursor to these hormones. In a chain reaction, cholesterol is first converted into pregnenolone and then into all the other steroidal hormones. When we become deficient in these hormones as we age, the body responds by producing more cholesterol in order to increase steroid hormone synthesis. By taking cholesterol-lowering drugs, we oppose the corrective measures instituted by the body. Perhaps this is why the long-term, drug-induced lowering of cholesterol has yielded no real advantages.

Dzugan and Smith found that by replacing the steroidal hormones lost to ageing (pregnenolone, dihydroepiandrosterone, progesterone, estrogen and total testosterone), all the trialists experienced a significant reduction in blood cholesterol levels comparable to the magnitude of cholesterol lowering normally to be expected from the statins.

The study also describes how a deficiency in these important hormones is the underlying cause of many disorders associated with normal ageing, including rising cholesterol levels and increased risk for heart attacks. It also brings to the fore the fact that hormone replacement therapy, until now mainly used by women, is equally important in men. It could well be that many of the adverse effects once ascribed to cholesterol were in fact manifestations of the harmful effects of hormonal imbalances.

A typical example is the strong association between testosterone levels in males and heart attack risk. A shortage of testosterone has been shown to be an important cause of heart muscle weakness[231], and one study has shown that there is a stronger correlation between testosterone blood levels and heart disease than between blood cholesterol levels and heart attacks[232].

In some people who have suffered a heart attack and who also have elevated cholesterol levels, correction of the cholesterol levels will not reduce the risk of a further heart attack because the real culprit is the low testosterone level.

During this study, the average serum total cholesterol levels dropped by 25,6% (from 6,52 to 4,82 mmol/l). These are significant reductions, comparable to or even better than what may be achieved by means of the statins.

The authors show that a person with a normal cholesterol level who had undergone the average age-associated elevation of 1,56 mmol/l over time is as much at risk as the person with a high cholesterol level who had undergone the same elevation. This explains why at least 60% of people with normal blood cholesterol values have heart attacks.

This study is the first of its kind, and it will have to be repeated by others before it is widely accepted. Nevertheless, its implications are that the age-associated hormone decline and resulting hormonal imbalances are among the risk factors for a heart attack and not the associated cholesterol values. This would explain many of the anomalies in the relationship between cholesterol and heart disease.

THE 'VITAMIN C' THEORY OF HEART DISEASE

Vitamin C plays a vital role in the biosynthesis of collagen and elastin, the connective tissue components present in artery walls. If there is a deficiency of vitamin C, the connective tissue structures in the artery walls become defective, creating the opportunity for the deposition of cholesterol and other deposits. These ultimately lead to the narrowing of arteries and the formation of blood clots.

Prof Linus Pauling, two-time Nobel prize winner and one of the most brilliant scientists of the 20th century, first focused attention on the benefits of high-dose vitamin C for the treatment of the common cold. Matthias Rath, a professor of medicine in Germany, also conducted research on vitamin C. He later joined Linus Pauling where together they formulated their vitamin C theory of heart disease in the early 1990s.

Elevated Lpa levels[233] in the body are seen only in those species, like us, that have lost the ability to make their own vitamin C.

For this reason, Lpa is regarded as a surrogate for vitamin C, and is made in the body in times of dietary vitamin C deficiency to prevent the inevitable vascular degeneration.

The process of atherosclerosis begins with a lesion (tear) in the artery wall, pointing to weakness in the artery wall and therefore defective collagen synthesis. Once such a lesion has formed, further development of the process of atherosclerosis consists of attempts by the body to heal the initial lesions, and this involves the deposition of fibrinogen/fibrin, thus creating the conditions for the formation of a blood clot. Cholesterol and other compounds that ultimately lead to the build-up of plaques are also deposited.

Plaques are not randomly distributed in the vascular system but are limited to those areas near to the heart with the highest pressure; here weaknesses and breaks linked to faulty synthesis of collagen are most likely to appear. Thus plaques are only formed at sites where underlying vascular weaknesses are most vulnerable to the formation of lesions. Veins, where pressures are much lower, generally do not suffer plaque deposits.

If the initial events in the formation of a vascular lesion were primarily determined by some other 'toxin' such as homocysteine or oxidised cholesterol, there would be a more random distribution of plaque in the vascular system. There is no reason why these 'toxins' should attack only sites in the vicinity of the heart.

According to the Pauling-Rath theory, this does not mean that factors such as oxidised cholesterol and homocysteine are not involved in heart disease (they clearly are), but that they play their role mainly after the initial lesions have been formed as a result of the vitamin C–Lpa mechanism.

The process of plaque formation is thus related to scurvy, where weaknesses and breaks in the micro-vasculature occur as a result of a deficiency of vitamin C.

The Pauling-Rath theory proposes that humans have lost their ability to produce vitamin C through the centuries due to altered living and dietary conditions, and therefore developed the capacity to produce Lpa as a surrogate for vitamin C to prevent fatal vascular bleeding which might have eliminated the species.

THE LYSINE CONNECTION

Lysine is one of the essential amino acids and a building block of the structural protein collagen. In the process of attaching to the vascular wall in an attempt to seal the leaky vascular wall, the Lpa molecule is known to attach itself to the lysine sites in the collagen matrix of the injured artery.

For this reason Pauling suggested that by providing extra lysine in the blood to compete with the lysine-binding sites on the collagen molecules, the Lpa molecules would be prevented from attaching to vascular collagen molecules, thus preventing plaque build-up.

The combination of vitamin C and lysine used in the treatment and prevention of heart disease has been shown to be dramatically effective in recent case studies. There have also been indications that existing cardiovascular disease may be reversed in this same way.

Proline is another amino acid that selectively inhibits binding of Lpa to the vascular wall. There are therefore three primary Lpa binding inhibitor substances: vitamin C, L-lysine and L-proline.

THE ROLE OF VITAMIN C IN HEART DISEASE

In dealing with the treatment and prevention of heart disease, it is vitally important to understand that the process of plaque building in the artery wall is essentially a healing process in response to primary lesions.

If the artery wall is repeatedly and constantly damaged, the healing process may progress to the point where narrowing of the arteries becomes clinically visible (angina pectoris). If continued, this process may culminate in a heart attack.

If the coronary arteries are only partly occluded so that the heart muscle suffers from a non-fatal lack of blood and oxygen, the condition is called angina pectoris. The medical approach is to perform a coronary bypass operation.

Yet, when the cardiologists cut or otherwise damage the arterial wall, it should come as no surprise that new scab formation takes place, which results in accelerated atherosclerosis. Most patients who have had a coronary bypass have to undergo another operation in two or three years' time. By cutting away the worst affected parts, the basic disease process has not been addressed and will continue unless the patient changes his or her lifestyle and diet (reduce refined carbohydrates, more vitamin C and more vitamins to combat homocysteine).

Any therapy that unnaturally interferes with this healing process is bound to fail in the end. The only effective treatment is to remove the basic cause, the arterial lesions that are formed as a result of a chronic vitamin C deficiency.

One reason why many cardiologists do not consider the evidence of vitamin therapy is that not enough full-scale clinical trials have been done. However, Pauling considers such trials unnecessary since virtually every patient treated in this way has responded dramatically. There is little doubt, though, that when a sponsor is willing to fund the necessary costly clinical trials without the prospect of financial rewards (since vitamin C cannot be patented), Pauling will be proven right.

Clinical evidence for the vitamin C theory

In the meantime, consider the clinical evidence already available in support of the Pauling-Rath theory.

Double blind, placebo-controlled trials are regarded by the medical profession as the 'gold standard' when it comes to proof, because of all study designs they have the smallest opportunity for bias and error. However, such trials are prohibitively expensive, which is why the available clinical information involves observational studies.

In his work Linus Pauling soon saw that patients responded well to the vitamin C + lysine therapy. Virtually every patient with heart disease does respond, and the results are there for everyone to see.

Vitamin C supplementation has been shown to improve arterial dilation 'stretch' response in people with chronic heart failure. This condition is associated with the stretch capacity of the vascular endothelial lining. Another clinical study has confirmed the favourable effects of vitamin C on the arterial wall lesion activity in people with coronary heart disease[64].

Supporting evidence of the effects of vitamin C in the prevention of heart disease is provided by the results of a Finnish population study in which it was found that a dietary intake of 200–500 mg per day of vitamin C correlated with a heart attack reduction of 50% and an increased life expectancy of six years[65].

This study, which was published in 1997, evaluated 1 605 randomly selected men (42–60 years old) with no previous history of heart disease for a period of five years. After adjusting for other confounding variables, men who were deficient in vitamin C had 3,5 times more heart attacks than those who were not deficient. The scientists concluded that 'vitamin C deficiency, as assessed by low plasma ascorbate concentration, is a risk factor for coronary heart disease'[66].

A 2001 Cambridge study involving 19 000 people looked at serum vitamin C levels and how long people lived. People who had the lowest levels of vitamin C were found to be twice as likely to die compared to those with the highest vitamin C levels[67].

A VITAMIN C REGIME

In practical terms, the Pauling-Rath vitamin C theory proposes a regime of 1 000–3 000 mg of vitamin C a day, to strengthen and heal blood vessels and to lower blood Lpa levels.

They also propose 3–5 g of L-lysine daily, to inhibit binding of Lpa and fibrinogen to vascular walls, and 2–4 g of L-proline a day for the same purpose.

Unlike the other drugs mentioned earlier in this chapter, there are no health risks associated with the treatment.

OTHER RISK FACTORS FOR HEART ATTACKS

It is unlikely that the final solution to the problem of CAD will come in the form of a single approach such as cholesterol lowering. CAD is without doubt a multifactorial problem, which may have to be dealt with on the basis of a multifaceted approach.

The nature of the problem is also such that it is quite possible that if any one of these measures is neglected, the others will become less effective. In addition to increased exercise, weight reduction, reduced intake of refined foods, and cholesterol lowering, blood levels of homocysteine, lipoprotein a, blood antioxidants, fibrinogen and hidden vascular infections will need to be considered.

It is important to realise that all the known risk factors for heart disease (including cholesterol) can account for less than 50% of the total risk.

An elevated LDL level is only one of the risk factors, and perhaps not even the most important one. Every heart patient should be investigated for the presence of at least the following risk factors, in addition to cholesterol: raised levels of homocysteine, elevated levels of C-reactive protein, fibrinogen, triglycerides, lipoprotein a and hormonal imbalances.

Raised levels of homocysteine

Homocysteine is an amino acid derived from the essential sulphur-containing amino acid methionine during its metabolic conversion in the body. Methionine acts as a methyl donor (it provides one-carbon units called methyl groups) in a variety of biosynthetic pathways. After losing its methyl group, methionine is converted into homocysteine, which then appears in the blood.

Homocysteine is extremely harmful to the vascular wall, which is why there are two mechanisms operative in the blood for the control of elevated homocysteine levels.

Both mechanisms are dependent on micronutrients.

In the first, homocysteine is reconverted back into methionine and other harmless products with the aid of vitamins B6, B12 and folic acid.

In the second, homocysteine is reconverted back into methionine in a biochemical reaction involving trimethyl glycine (betaine).

C-reactive protein

Some heart patients and stroke victims develop vascular diseases without an indication of any known cause, but what all these patients have in common are mildly elevated levels of a protein called C-reactive protein (CRP). Significantly raised levels of CRP in the blood have been used for many years as a method to indicate the existence of a focus of inflammation somewhere in the body.

Fibrinogen

Fibrinogen is a blood protein produced in the liver, and it forms an integral part of the blood clotting mechanism.

During the formation of a blood clot, fibrinogen is first converted into fine strands of fibrin; these form a blood clot when blood platelets become entangled in the fibrin strands. The terminal event in a heart attack is usually the formation of a blood clot at a site in the vascular wall where a plaque has developed.

Several studies have demonstrated a close association between blood fibrinogen levels and risk for heart attacks. The risk increases significantly when blood fibrinogen levels are above 3,5 g/l. Blood fibrinogen levels may be lowered by taking vitamin A (20 000 IU), fish oil (4–6 g) and vitamin C (2 000 mg) supplements.

Triglycerides

Fats in the blood are transported in the form of protein complexes in which long-chain fatty acid molecules are joined to glycol, hence the name triglycerides (TG). Blood levels of TG are critically influenced by diet, and the best way in which to control TG is by reducing the intake of refined carbohydrates in the diet.

Risk for heart attacks increase when blood TG levels are above 1,0 mmol/l.

Lipoprotein a

Lipoprotein a (Lpa) is a blood lipid that is closely related to LDL. In fact, Lpa is produced in the body from LDL (the 'bad' cholesterol) by the addition of just one protein molecule (Apo a). It is an adhesive glycoprotein (contains sugar residues which make it sticky) that attaches to the fibrous proteins around vascular walls, thus sealing the leaks that have occurred as a result of defective collagen synthesis. High levels (above 300 mg/l) are associated with an increased risk for heart attacks. High doses (2 000 mg) of N-Acetylcysteine may be used to reduce elevated levels of Lpa.

MAKING THE RIGHT DECISIONS

Coronary artery disease and therefore heart attacks are multifactorial conditions in which more than one factor may be involved.

The most important risk factors are raised levels of homocysteine, abnormal blood cholesterol values and vitamin C deficiency, although the importance of cholesterol in relation to heart risk has been grossly overemphasised. This perhaps explains why after all these years of heart disease awareness campaigns and treatment, no clear benefit to the person with heart disease has emerged. Death as a result of a heart attack remains the most common cause of death in the Western world.

CHAPTER TWO

OSTEOPOROSIS

OSTEOPOROSIS – THE CALCIUM BANDWAGON

Osteoporosis is an extremely common condition, yet so many people, including those who suffer from it, appear to know very little about the disease.

If you want to live a full and active life, it is essential that you make the right, informed decisions about preventing and treating this disorder as you grow older. Osteoporosis is nearly always a companion of old age, and it is not only debilitating but in many cases life threatening. The condition does far more than cause bone fragility and occasional pains and aches.

The overall lifetime risk of a woman suffering from a fracture is 40%, which is more than the combined risk of getting breast, ovarian and endometrial cancer.

Successful treatment and prevention strategies are hampered by the fact that some outdated and outright wrong beliefs are still widely circulating. The most important of these myths (and you'll hear it from doctors, too) is the assumption that you can do nothing about the condition, and that to prevent it you need only take estrogen and calcium supplements and drink a lot of milk.

Such advice is not only wrong and achieves nothing by way of preventing the disease, but it may be harmful in the long term. The truth is that, in general, calcium supplements should never be taken alone but always in combination with magnesium and other minerals (see page 46), which are usually more important than calcium. (However, an intake of less than 500 mg of calcium a day probably does necessitate calcium supplementation anyway.)

OSTEOPOROSIS BASICS

A certain amount of bone loss occurs naturally as we age (type 1 osteoporosis), because of declining hormone levels, lack of exercise and poor nutrition. It is typically caused by the loss of trabecular bone, the porous material that occurs in the inner bone. Normally bone loss for women is 10% of total bone mass per decade, which takes place from the age of 30; men lose around 6% per decade. This means that by the time a woman reaches 80, she will have lost 50% of her bone mass.

Bone loss increases in the postmenopausal years, and may be as high as 4–5% per year during menopause and a number of years thereafter. When this occurs, there is an increased risk of fractures, mainly vertebral, distal forearm and ankle fractures.

Secondary osteoporosis occurs later in life and is associated with a loss of cortical (the outer shell-like covering of bones) as well as trabecular bone, and frequently results in hip fractures.

Different lifestyle and personal factors may accelerate the process of osteoporosis. These include, among others, a family history of osteoporosis, hormonal deficiencies (estrogen, progesterone), drugs (particularly corticoids), smoking, lack of exercise and mineral deficiencies.

Osteoporotic fractures should be avoided at all costs because they have serious long-term consequences. Ordinary fractures in younger people are not normally a threat to health, but in the older person with osteoporosis it is more serious; this is because the bone shatters and splinters, so the healing process is retarded and complicated. Most people do not die of osteoporosis itself but rather from the complications that result. Less than 50% of those with this type of fracture will be able to return to their previous level of functioning.

If you ask an uninformed doctor for advice on how to prevent osteoporosis, you are likely to be told to take calcium supplements, drink at least a litre of milk per day and, if you are a postmenopausal woman, to take hormones in the form of Premarin or a combination of Premarin and synthetic progestogen (see chapter 3).

Each element of this advice (prevention and treatment) is seriously wrong, and may even be harmful.

THE COMPOSITION OF BONE

Bone consists of a protein matrix (20%) onto which minerals are deposited during the bone-building process. These minerals are mainly calcium, magnesium, zinc and a number of microminerals, each of which has a specific function in the formation and maintenance of bone.

The matrix consists of type-T collagen and small quantities of non-collagenous and glycoproteins, each of which serves a specific purpose although full details are not yet known. Collagen is the body's main structural protein, while glycoproteins are proteins linked to sugar molecules. The non-collagenous proteins consist mostly of the protein osteocalcin and the mineral-transporting protein osteronectin.

THE ROLE OF CALCIUM

There can be no doubt that calcium is an important bone mineral, even though it is not the only bone mineral.

Generations of doctors have taught that calcium supplementation and drinking milk are ways to prevent osteoporosis. In addition, a decade-long intensive campaign to promote the consumption of milk products has convinced many millions, including doctors, that calcium supplementation bestows perfect bone health, especially upon women and growing children. There is no doubt that milk is a good source of calcium, but it is not a good source for building bone because it lacks other vital minerals such as magnesium. The advice about milk was given solely on the basis that calcium (quantity-wise) is the principal mineral in bone. This does not mean that giving calcium in isolation or drinking milk will promote bone formation.

What we do have is evidence that bone loss is accelerated if calcium intake is lower than 500 mg a day (the average person eating a good diet takes in around 800 mg of calcium). What is less certain is whether increasing calcium intake to above this level on its own will effectively prevent or retard bone loss.

Despite years of calcium supplementation, total incidence as well as age-specific incidence of osteoporosis is sharply on the increase[86]. Today osteoporosis affects more than 20 million Americans, with nearly two million fractures a year (responsible for suffering, loss of life, and huge costs in excess of $3,5 billion annually). In South Africa around 3–4 million people suffer from the disease.

Osteoporosis is more prevalent in the developed world, where the intake of milk products is high[87]. In many of the developing countries, the staple plant foods contain much more magnesium than calcium. For example, maize provides 830 mg of magnesium and only 124 mg of calcium per 10 000 kJ, resulting in a magnesium/calcium ratio of 6:7. In contrast, the ratio in milk is only 0:11[88].

Bone formation cannot take place in the absence of adequate quantities of magnesium (around 300–500 mg a day). No experimental evidence has ever been presented to clearly demonstrate that high doses of calcium (more than 1 000 mg a day), taken over long periods, can prevent osteoporosis. Some people, on the advice of their doctors, take up to 1 500 mg a day, which may be harmful (see below).

Nevertheless, calcium is a vital bone mineral. When supplements are necessary (when your daily intake is less than 500 mg), no more than 500–800 mg of elemental calcium should be taken, and this should be given in the correct, absorbable form.

A good form is calcium-citrate malate (a complex of calcium with the organic acids citric acid and malic acid). Although calcium glycinate (calcium salt of the amino acid glycine) is somewhat better absorbed, it is also more expensive, so it is more economical and equally effective to take more (20%) of the calcium-citrate malate. The worst forms are the oxides and carbonates. These are not only poorly absorbed, but have the added disadvantage of neutralising stomach acid, which is vitally important for mineral metabolism[92].

THE PRINCIPLE OF SYNERGISM

Calcium is not a drug. It is an important nutrient, and nutrients never act in isolation.

Many of the clinical studies on nutrients have been conducted with single nutrients, and invariably such studies have yielded information that was of little real value. The clinical response to any particular nutrient is largely dependent on the relative status of the individual or group, with respect to the other synergistic nutrients for the particular nutrient tested.

Results obtained from supplementation with single nutrients are often a better reflection of this relative status than of the actual effects of the nutrient tested. The results obtained with calcium supplementation bone density studies are a good example; some studies have found that calcium supplementation increases bone density, while others have not been able to confirm this.

This has nothing to do with the methodology or the integrity of the researchers – it simply reflects the overall mineral status with respect to the other synergistic minerals concerned in the study populations used.

Clinical researchers are often doctors with a sound training in pharmacology but with little (or no) training in nutritional science. The result is that nutrients are evaluated in much the same way as individual drugs.

In pharmacology, it is frowned upon to use more than one drug at a time – this is often known as 'shotgun therapy'. But this is precisely the way nutrients act, and therefore the way in which they should be used.

There should no longer be any doubt that calcium, on its own, cannot build a shred of bone, because bone consists of many minerals (magnesium, silicon, fluoride, zinc, copper, boron, manganese and phosphorus), each with a specific function. In the process of bone building, these minerals and many other nutrients are required.

If any one of these is in short supply, and this is often the case, the process of bone formation will be retarded. Depending on the severity of the deficiency, this may even lead to overall loss of bone, in spite of adequate intake of calcium.

Results obtained from calcium supplementation studies have frequently been confounded by the body's inherent ability to adapt to low calcium intakes by means of increased absorption and reduced excretion[94]. Calcium retention is also critically influenced by magnesium status.

MAGNESIUM

Of all the factors that support the skeleton, the calcium/magnesium ratio is perhaps the most important – and it is an excellent example of the interdependence of nutrients.

When blood magnesium levels decline, the kidneys readjust the calcium/magnesium ratio by excreting more calcium, and vice versa when magnesium levels rise. Thus supplementation with magnesium is one way of improving calcium retention[95]. Supplementation with magnesium (even high levels) does not suppress calcium absorption[96] as is sometimes claimed.

For preventing and possibly reversing osteoporosis in practice, magnesium may be even more important than calcium[97] – and it is often more deficient in Western diets than is calcium.

In one study, magnesium supplements (without calcium) were given to post-menopausal women with signs of progressing osteoporosis. After two years, there was either an increase in bone density or an arrest of further bone loss in 87% of the patients[98]. The results of another study published in 1994 confirm that optimal bone formation cannot take place in the absence of magnesium, no matter how much calcium is taken.

MAGNESIUM, MINERAL DISTRIBUTION AND EXCESS CALCIUM

Bone density is determined not only by the type and quantities of minerals absorbed, but also by the distribution and ultimate fate of these nutrients in the body. Magnesium and vitamins K and D are important determinants of mineral distribution.

Magnesium has been shown to increase bone mineral density in men and women[99], achieved by increasing the retention of calcium in bone. A magnesium deficiency (a dietary intake of less than 200 mg a day and a blood level of less than 0,7 mmol/l) can cause bone to stop growing, as well as increase bone fragility and fractures[233].

A large percentage of the body's calcium is present in the skeleton, and the rest is present in the blood and tissues, including the artery walls. Accumulation of excessive quantities of calcium in the artery walls leads to a condition known as 'hardening of the arteries' or arteriosclerosis, often in the middle layers of the arteries. (Arteriosclerosis is to be distinguished from atherosclerosis, which refers to the accumulation of plaque, connective tissue and fatty deposits in the artery walls associated with an increased risk of heart disease and stroke.)

Hardening of the arteries in the middle layers of the arteries is not immediately visible and has nothing to do with fats or cholesterol. Sudden death from a heart attack is often associated with extensive calcification of the aorta, especially in young men.

Magnesium plays a pivotal role in the process of tissue calcification, and a prominent feature of magnesium deficiency is the deposition of calcium in certain tissues. Calcium excess leads to soft tissue calcification and this condition is aggravated in the presence of a magnesium deficiency[100]. Further studies have shown that excess calcium in the presence of low magnesium promotes deposition of calcium in the blood vessels, including the brain[101]. These observations are particularly significant at a time when amounts in excess of 1 000 mg daily of calcium are routinely given over long periods (for the treatment of osteoporosis) to people who are not monitored for a magnesium deficiency. Magnesium deficiency is extremely common[102] in the developed world where it has been shown that 80% of the population get considerably less than the recommended intake (RDA). Even the RDA, at 300 mg a day, has been considered to be too low. Most osteoporosis patients have very low magnesium levels[103].

VITAMIN K

In recent years, vitamin K has attracted considerable attention as a regulator of bone and tissue calcification, as it keeps calcium inside bones and out of arteries.

Vitamin K, in an enzymatic reaction, forms gammacarboxyglutamic acid (Gla), a derivative of the amino acid glutamic acid. Calcium-carrying proteins are formed when Gla is incorporated as one or more of the amino acids in their amino acid chains, and these protein molecules are able to hold on to calcium, thus forming a special type of chelate. After grabbing a calcium ion, the complex can move around and enter bone structures where the calcium can be deposited.

Under conditions of vitamin K deficiency calcium drifts out of bones and is then deposited in tissues in close proximity of the circulating blood, mainly the arteries.

The Gla protein called osteocalcin has been used as an indicator of bone formation in order to monitor bone loss or growth. What is not generally known is that this protein also requires vitamin K.

With a vitamin K deficiency, the risk of suffering a bone fracture increases[105] and one study found a relationship between decreased bone density and low levels of vitamin K in men[106].

When taking anticoagulants like warfarin, remember that they work by suppressing vitamin K activity in cells. Broccoli, Brussels sprouts, cauliflower and lettuce are good sources of vitamin K. Interestingly, vitamin K has for many years been considered to be important only in the process of blood clotting. It is now clear that it has other major functions in the body, including that of bone formation.

VITAMIN D3

Vitamin D3, like vitamin K, has functions that go well beyond those traditionally assigned to it. Some of these functions are hormone-like in effect.

Vitamin D is a steroid-like molecule that occurs in different forms in nature; vitamin D3 is the form naturally present in humans, also known as cholecalciferol. In South Africa, young people do not have to take supplements if they have a reasonable amount of exposure to sunshine, but the elderly need to, for optimal health.

First indications of such an effect were obtained from human studies that showed that vitamin D3 plus calcium improved bone density, while calcium alone did not. The results could not be explained on the basis of calcium concentration alone[107]. Clearly vitamin D3 has effects other than improving mineral absorption.

Studies are now available that consistently show the vitamin's hormone-like action by directing calcium (and presumably other minerals) to the bone and by suppressing parathyroid action, thus suppressing demineralisation of bone.

These results suggest that, in future, osteoporosis patients should consider supplementation with higher than usual doses of vitamin D3 against a background of maintenance intake of calcium.

OTHER MINERALS

In order to use calcium in the process of bone building, the body needs adequate quantities of at least seven minerals (zinc, boron, silicon, copper, fluoride, manganese and phosphorus) and vitamin D3, in addition to magnesium and vitamin K[108].

Zinc deficiency causes a reduction in osteoblast (bone-forming cell) activity along with impaired collagen formation. Collagen forms part of the matrix onto which minerals such as calcium and magnesium are precipitated in the process of bone formation.

Copper deficiency prevents cross-linking and therefore mechanical strength in the matrix proteins collagen and elastin.

Manganese deficiency suppresses biosynthesis of matrix mucopolysaccharides, which serve as structural support in the body as well as acting as bone-building catalysts in the maintenance and building of the organic bone matrix.

Thirty years of clinical trials have shown that the trace mineral boron is essential for healthy bones and joints[109]. Boron regulates estrogen and testosterone metabolism and reduces excretion of calcium and magnesium. In response to boron, bone loss is suppressed and estrogen and testosterone levels rise in postmenopausal women when magnesium levels are low. Boron thus prevents excessive urinary excretion of calcium and magnesium.

Giving a calcium-only supplement to such patients will not help to either prevent or treat osteoporosis.

BONE DENSITY AND VITAMIN C

The organic matrix in bone – which consists largely of collagen and elastin fibres – is the structural framework that holds the minerals together.

The overall process of collagen synthesis comprises several steps, and vitamin C is involved in each of them. This explains so much about human vitamin C requirements that is so seldom appreciated. Only 1–2% of the human body consists of collagen, a significant percentage of which is present in the collagenous matrix proteins, and all of which has to undergo constant regeneration.

This requires relatively large amounts of vitamin C, as the vitamin is consumed in the regeneration process. Clearly then, adequate quantities of vitamin C are a prerequisite for the healthy regeneration of bones.

PROGESTERONE

Estrogens such as Premarin (see chapter 3) are widely prescribed to help combat post-menopausal osteoporosis, but their value is limited by the fact that the anti-osteoporosis effect of estrogens wane after a number of years. There are two types of bone cells involved in maintaining bone density. Osteoclasts are bone cells that break down bone by dissolving the bone minerals. The other type of bone cells, osteoblasts, form new bone.

When the activity of these two types of cells are in equilibrium, bone density is maintained. Various biological molecules are able to activate either type of bone cell and in this manner affect bone density.

Estrogens inhibit osteoclastic activity and thus suppress bone loss – this is why they can retard but not reverse osteoporosis[111], and this is what happens in the postmenopausal woman on estrogen therapy.

Progesterone is a hormone that opposes estrogen action in many ways, and this is also the case with bone metabolism. Estrogen works best in combination with progesterone and cannot protect against bone loss when progesterone is absent.

Progesterone, on the other hand, can cause a true reversal of osteoporosis even in patients who do not use estrogen[112].

Clearly, a combination of estrogen and progesterone would be more effective than estrogen alone, since this also mimics what happens naturally in the premenopausal woman. Synthetic progestogens appear to have a much weaker effect than natural progesterone on bone density (see page 60).

HOMOCYSTEINE AND OSTEOPOROSIS

Homocysteine is an unnatural amino acid (it does not occur in food) that is formed in the body when there is a deficiency of vitamins B6, B12 and folic acid. It is a serious risk factor for heart disease and stroke (see chapter 1).

A review of studies published since 1972 reveals that homocysteine may accelerate osteoporosis by interfering with the process of protein bone matrix synthesis in a way that results in the formation of a defective bone matrix[113].

A study, done in 1985, showed that supplemental folic acid (which reduces blood homocysteine levels) helps protect against osteoporosis by protecting the bone matrix against the toxic effects of homocysteine[114].

Anyone who is concerned about their long-term health should know their blood homocysteine levels. If the level is above 8,0 mmol/l, additional vitamins (as indicated previously) should be taken[19].

THE WAY AHEAD

The time has come to rethink our approach to the problem of osteoporosis treatment and prevention.

Certainly the 'calcium-only' approach of the past decades is no longer tenable, as it assumes that all the other vital nutrients required for the formation of healthy bones are present in adequate amounts.

In future, supplementation programmes should be aimed not only at supplying all the nutrients required for bone formation, but also those involved in the process of mineral distribution.

The good news is that osteoporosis is both preventable and treatable. Most elderly women have undergone a degree of bone loss, depending on genetic disposition and lifestyle. If you are over 50, it is time to assess your bone status. The best procedure is to have a bone scan (with the aid of your doctor) using dual X-ray technology (DEXA). This test unfortunately only reveals bone loss once a significant amount of bone has already been lost. If you need to know how much bone you have lost, have a bone mass density test conducted.

SIGNS OF BONE LOSS

If you have more than three of these signs (featured below and opposite), you need a full evaluation of your bone mineral status:
➤ **leg cramps (also indicate a possible magnesium deficiency)**
➤ **heavy plaque formation on teeth**
➤ **receding gum lines**
➤ **tendency toward kidney stones (indicates accelerated mobilisation of minerals from bone)**
➤ **loose teeth**
➤ **osteoarthritic changes in joints with pain and tenderness**

- ➤ back pain which may appear suddenly
- ➤ fractures that form easily
- ➤ round shoulders
- ➤ prominent abdomen
- ➤ neck inclined forward
- ➤ loss of height
- ➤ occasional leg pain

RISK FACTORS FOR OSTEOPOROSIS
- ➤ Women are more at risk than men because of their hormonal patterns, but by the age of 65–70, men and women lose bone at the same rate. However, at this stage women have already lost more bone than men and are therefore still at greater risk
- ➤ A history of osteoporosis in the family
- ➤ Smoking increases the risk considerably
- ➤ Alcohol stimulates the osteoclasts (cells that break down bone) and therefore increases bone loss. Alcohol also promotes excretion of magnesium, which is much needed for healthy bones
- ➤ Some prescription drugs, such as cortisone, thyroid hormones, anticoagulants and antacids, have a particularly strong negative effect on osteoporosis. However, use these drugs only when it is really necessary and then for the shortest possible time
- ➤ A diet high in processed foods and refined sugars
- ➤ An excessive intake of protein (especially animal protein)
- ➤ Lack of exercise. (Do regular weight bearing exercise – running and walking)
- ➤ Estrogen deficiency in women and testosterone deficiency in men are also risk factors – see chapter 3 for the best type of hormone replacements

A SUGGESTED SUPPLEMENT REGIME
- ➤ Calcium: 500–800 mg (chelated)
- ➤ Magnesium: 400–500 mg (chelated)
- ➤ Boron: 6–9 mg (chelated)
- ➤ Zinc: 30 mg (chelated)
- ➤ Silicon: 30 mg

➤ Vitamin D3: 400–600 IU (10–15 mcg)
➤ Vitamin C: 1 000–3 000 mg
➤ Vitamin K: 150–200 mcg
➤ Multivitamin/mineral supplement (with microminerals and vitamin B6: 10 mg, vitamin B12: 100 mcg and folic acid: 2 mg)
➤ Estrogen supplements (postmenopausal women). Estrogens should be used in conjunction with natural progesterone cream
➤ Use one of the following as advised by your doctor: Estriol 2–8 mg (tablets); or Estriol cream (as directed). Use in combination with progesterone cream
➤ Soy isoflavone extract: to supply 100–150 mg of soy isoflavones

CHAPTER THREE

HRT ALERT

If you're interested in health, you're likely to develop an ear that's sensitive to new rumblings in the health arena. So I immediately realised that something was afoot when my telephone began ringing more often than usual, with calls from women concerned about the safety of hormone replacement therapy (HRT) and especially estrogen replacement therapy (ERT), as currently practised by the medical profession.

I am a medical scientist and not a gynaecologist or medical practitioner, so my task is neither to prescribe nor diagnose but rather to inform patients and doctors on the latest developments in the medical field that may affect their health.

However, I do know that for the past few years, women   especially those in the menopausal and postmenopausal years – have been nurturing doubts about the safety of the prescribed hormone replacement drugs, in spite of assurances by their doctors. Today that trickle of doubting women has become a flood.

This concern was precipitated in mid-2002 by a number of reports in the popular press about the abrupt termination of a major clinical trial in America, because of the higher incidence of cancer in the group being treated with Prempro, the estrogen/progestin drug. It is ethical practice in clinical trials to terminate them if the drug in question turns out to have serious side effects, or even if the drug turns out to be effective (so as not to compromise the participants not taking the drug).

One of the major objectives of hormone therapy is to replace vital female hormones (estrogen and progesterone) pharmacologically. These hormones are produced mainly in the ovaries, and during and after menopause their production declines, causing relative deficiencies that are manifested as the many unpleasant symptoms associated with the menopause.

When more than one hormone (such as estrogen plus progesterone) is replaced, it is known as hormone replacement therapy (HRT), and when only estrogen is replaced, it is known as estrogen replacement therapy (ERT).

The drug in the trial above was a combination of conjugated estrogens and a synthetic progestogen (not to be confused with the natural hormone progesterone). In this context, 'conjugated' means that the estrogen combines naturally with glucuronic acid and other carrier molecules in the horse.

The progestin in the drug Prempro was medroxyprogesterone acetate, a commonly used synthetic progestogen, which differs in many ways from the natural progesterone.

The conjugated estrogen component in Prempro consisted of conjugated horse estrogens containing conjugated estrone and other estrogenic compounds present in horse urine (similar to those present in the popular drug Premarin).

At the time of the Prempro trials, Premarin was being used, on medical prescription, by six million women in the United States alone.

The clinical trial noted above formed a part of the Women's Health Initiative (WHI), a study programme initiated in 1998 in the United States to study diseases in women. This particular trial involved 8 506 women (aged between 50 and 79 years) in the treatment group and 8 102 in the control group (who were on no form of treatment at all), and was scheduled to run until 2005. However, it was abruptly stopped in 2002, because the Data and Safety Monitoring Board decided that the overall health risks exceeded the benefits. Specifically, they found an unacceptable level of invasive breast cancer among the patients in the study using the particular combination of estrogen and progestogen.

In addition, the board found that women in the treatment group had a significantly increased risk of heart attacks and strokes. This contrasts with medical teaching and practice over the previous 30 years, during which millions of women had been treated in this manner.

The table on the opposite page, published in the *Journal of the American Medical Association*[68] summarises the results (cases per 1 000 women per year):

	HRT	PLACEBO	DIFFERENCE
Breast cancer	3,8	3,0	+26%
Heart disease	3,7	3,9	+23%
Stroke	2,9	2,1	+38%
Blood clots	2,6	1,3	+100%
Hip fractures	1,0	1,5	-33%
Colon cancer	1,0	1,6	-37%

In other words, 26% more women taking the drug will develop breast cancer compared to a group of women not taking the drug; 23% more will develop heart disease; 38% more will develop stroke and 100% more will develop blood clots. However, 33% fewer will develop hip fractures and 37% fewer will develop colon cancer.

This study, when taken together with the results of many smaller, previous studies, establishes that hormone replacement therapy based on conjugated horse estrogens (such as Premarin) and taken together with synthetic progestogen (such as in Prempro) increases the risk of breast cancer. It is not surprising, then, that members of the public have reacted with alarm, and there has certainly been a major move away from horse estrogens in the medical profession.

One of the arguments in favour of HRT, used by the medical profession in the past, was that it resulted in reduced risk of heart disease. Doctors noted that while the risk of cancer did exist, such a risk was small and offset by the advantage of reducing heart attacks (the latter being far more prevalent among women of this age group than cancer).

These arguments have now been shown to be incorrect.

The relatively large increase in the incidence of stroke is unexpected and alarming, and is something to be considered when deciding on a supplementation programme. The relatively large decreases in hip fractures and colon cancer are a bonus.

The decision to terminate the trial must have been a shock to many, although to people in the field of natural medicine, the results were not such a surprise at all. Before this study, there had been at least 50 other, smaller, case-control studies that collectively pointed to the dangers associated with hormone supplements when substances such as horse estrogens are used. Synthesised estrogens, as opposed to horse estrogens, are less risky, provided that bio-identical hormones are used in the correct ratios.

WHAT IS PREMARIN?

Premarin consists of a mixture of 'conjugated horse estrogens' or 'conjugated equine estrogens (CEE)'. As implied by the name, Premarin is obtained, by suitable extraction procedures, from the urine of pregnant mares. 'Conjugated' means that the estrogen molecules in the product are chemically joined to carrier molecules such as glucuronic acid.

This happens in the animal, presumably to convert the water-insoluble steroids into more water-soluble products, which can be more readily excreted in the urine. Initially when these extracts were first studied for the purpose of developing a product that would be suitable for human use, it was shown that the estrogen component in the product consisted of the following ten estrogens:

➤ 17-beta-estradiol
➤ 17-alpha-estradiol
➤ estrone
➤ 17-beta-dihydroequilenin
➤ 17-alpha-dihydroequilenin
➤ 17-beta-dihydroequilin
➤ equilin
➤ delta 8,9-dehydroestrone sulphate
➤ equilenin
➤ estriol

Since then, advancements in analytical technology have revealed that the above 10 estrogens only make up 40% of the hormonal component of Premarin, and an additional 200 compounds have been identified including androgens (male hormones) and progesterone derivatives.

Most of these compounds do not occur in humans. Moreover, different types of estrogen have different effects in different tissues.

Most people believe that Premarin simply consists of conjugated forms of estradiol and estrone, the natural hormones present in human serum. This is not so, and the complexity of the product may be the cause of the toxic effects that studies into conjugated estrogen (CEE) have now revealed.

The Premarin estrogens are in no way equal or bio-identical to the natural human hormones estradiol, estrone and estriol.

This is also the reason for the large number of side effects experienced by women on CEE supplements (estrogen supplementation therapy or EST) whether the estrogen component is combined with a synthetic progestogen (HRT) or not.

Internationally, Premarin is sold as an estrogen supplement (estrogen replacement therapy or ERT). Prempro, the combination of conjugated estrogen and the synthetic progestin Provera, is known as hormone replacement therapy or HRT, which is prescribed if both hormones are thought to be deficient.

ESTROGEN ON ITS OWN

In July 2002 the National Cancer Institute (NCI) in the United States announced the results of its own study designed to investigate the relationship between horse estrogen supplements and ovarian cancer, a question that was considered to be controversial!

The NCI examined data from the Breast Cancer Detection Demonstration Project, a screening programme that studied a total of 44 241 postmenopausal women in 29 United States clinical centres over 19 years. The reason the study was conducted over such a long period was because it was known that breast cancer manifests only after eight or more years of horse estrogen supplementation.

The results showed that postmenopausal women who took horse estrogens for more than 10 years have a 60% higher increased risk of developing ovarian cancer than women who had never used horse estrogen.

The results also found that the chances of developing breast cancer increase sharply with the time a woman uses horse estrogen, which is in accord with the results of previous studies. The researchers concluded that a combination of horse estrogen plus progestin does not significantly increase the risk of ovarian cancer.

This latter finding could have offered some consolation, had it not been that the WHI study above found that this combination increased the risk of breast cancer. It seems, then, that there is little to be gained from the use of conjugated horse estrogens, whether these are used as such or in combination with synthetic progestogens.

Wyeth, the company that makes and markets Premarin, has circulated new guidelines to clinicians following the publication of the results of the two studies. The updated labels state, among other things, that:

➤ **These products are not indicated and should not be used to prevent coronary heart disease.**
➤ **Use should be limited to the shortest duration consistent with treatment goals and risks for the individual, and should be periodically re-evaluated.**
➤ **When used solely for the prevention of postmenopausal osteoporosis, alternative treatments should be carefully considered.**

The first point is directly contrary to previous medical opinion and practice, so indicates a significant turnaround. The second statement in fact says that these are dangerous products – don't use them! And the third statement is a carefully worded and ambiguous statement that simply means 'don't use these products for the prevention of osteoporosis'.

The results of these two trials come as bad news not only for the medical profession but also for the many women with serious menopausal problems, because there is no denying the considerable benefits that these preparations have in the treatment of many of the unpleasant symptoms of menopause.

WHAT IS ESTROGEN?

Estrogen is a collective term used loosely to refer to at least 20–30 hormone molecules with estrogenic activity in the human body. It is assumed that these all have different functions, although details are presently not known.

Estrogens are mainly produced in the ovaries in response to stimulation by two hormones called FSH and LH, produced in the pituitary gland. The three main estrogens in the blood are estradiol, estrone and estriol.

Estrogen levels rise and fall in a distinctive pattern during a woman's monthly cycle. During the menopause there is a gradual decline of estrogen production in the ovaries, which is accompanied by the usual unpleasant symptoms such as night sweats, hot flushes, sexual problems, hair loss, mood disorders, vaginal dryness and others.

Pharmacological administration of any one of these estrogens effectively reduces the symptoms, but unfortunately also has a variety of side effects such as increased incidence of cancer, especially after prolonged use (more than seven years).

The cancer risk associated with the use of estrogen supplements has been the subject of numerous studies over the last two or three decades. Some of these studies have yielded controversial results, but many have confirmed the increased cancer risk, especially of endometrial and breast cancer.

A study published in the *Journal of the American Medical Association* in 1998 found that supplementing with estrogen alone increased the breast cancer risk by 34%, compared to women taking no supplements, while the risk increases to 54% when estrogens are used in combination with a synthetic progestogen[69]. In this study there was also a 23% increased risk of heart attacks. These results were contrary to medical teaching and practice at that time.

A more recent study published in the same journal (2000) found that the risk for breast cancer increases by 10% for every five years on estrogen therapy, and even more when estrogens are combined with synthetic progestogens[70].

In the United States, there are 178 000 new cases of breast cancer a year, and this figure appears to be steadily on the increase. Every year 43 000 women die of breast cancer in the US, making it the second largest cause of cancer deaths. Today, one in every eight women in the US can expect to get breast cancer, which poses the question: how many of these deaths are the result of legally prescribed estrogen supplements?

WHY DOES THE MEDICAL PROFESSION STILL PROMOTE HRT?

Hormone Replacement Therapy (HRT) in its present form consists largely of those conjugated horse estrogens (Premarin) and these estrogens in combination with progestogens as discussed earlier. Why, then, do medical practitioners and gynaecologists persist in using them, despite the risks indicated in the medical literature?

One reason is because there is considerable pressure from menopausal women on their doctors to prescribe these drugs – there is no denying that supplementation with any one of the estrogens considerably alleviates many menopausal symptoms.

There is also considerable peer pressure: 'We prescribe them because it is standard medical practice and everyone else does,' say doctors. And, of course, there is considerable pressure by the manufacturing companies that actively promote the products, often exaggerating the benefits and minimising the risks. In discussions with medical doctors on the subject, I often received three standard answers: 'The risk is relatively small'; 'The benefits for the reduced heart attacks outweigh the cancer risk; and 'HRT significantly reduces the risk of osteoporosis.'

None of these answers are entirely correct, in the light of this evidence[69]. HRT does reduce the risk of osteoporosis to some extent. It is true that the bone loss in those on estrogen therapy is much reduced during the first 7–10 years of treatment, but the protective effect thereafter wanes, and those who had been on HRT then lose bone faster than those who had never taken the drug. In fact, bone loss starts at age 30 or so, when estrogen levels are still high, showing that estrogen is not the only factor that controls bone loss. In later life, when the danger of osteoporosis is the greatest, it makes no difference whether or not a woman took estrogens during and after the menopause[73].

HRT AND BREAST CANCER

In its present form and at its current dosage, HRT at best has temporary advantages only[74], while the risk of cancer is substantial. There are two types of invasive breast cancer: the non-lobular and the lobular.

The non-lobular (ductal) is the most common (75% of cases) and the least dangerous of the two. The lobular is less common (10–15% of cases) but much more dangerous and aggressive. As it is located in the deepest part of the breast, this type is more difficult to detect by physical examination and mammography. A recent study investigated the relative occurrence of the two types of breast cancer in women who had taken any form of HRT compared to those who had not[75].

The results, published in 2002, showed that the risk of breast cancer (both types) was 1,85 times higher in women who had used any form of HRT for more than 4,5 years. The risk for lobular cancer in the estrogen-only group was three times higher than in those who had not taken any form of HRT, while the estrogen plus progestin group had a four times higher risk of lobular cancer.

This study confirms the results of previous studies regarding the cancer risk in HRT users but shows that estrogen, and especially estrogen plus progestogen, increases the risk of the more dangerous type even more.

THE PROGESTOGENS

The progestogens are a group of synthetic chemicals with chemical structures similar but not identical to natural progesterone. Progesterone is produced monthly in the ovaries in the premenopausal woman after ovulation. Its production ceases at the end of the cycle if fertilisation did not take place; its function is otherwise to maintain a pregnancy, and is a strong stimulant of bone formation.

The progestogens were developed by drug companies in response to the demand for a progesterone derivative that can be administered orally – natural progesterone is broken down in the gut and during passage through the liver, so when taken orally in its natural form, it results in unpredictable blood levels. Although these progestogens do have some biological properties in common with natural progesterone, in other respects they differ considerably.

They also have many side effects, some of them serious: the possibility of birth defects; increased risk for breast cancer; increased risk for blood clots; and increased risk of fluid retention, rashes, weight gain and depression.

It is therefore not unexpected that some of these side effects showed up to a greater extent in studies when it was combined with Premarin than with Premarin alone.

IS THERE A SAFE LEVEL OF PREMARIN?

In most of the above studies, conjugated horse estrogens (such as in the drug Premarin) were used as a source of estrogen (rather than bio-identical hormones in the form of estradiol, estrone and estriol).

Many studies have been devoted to determining the relationship between Premarin intake and blood fats, especially LDL, HDL and blood cholesterol values. The results of these studies show that rising estrogen levels decrease LDL values while increasing HDL values. These are the changes that are commensurate with reduced cardiovascular risk and have been used in the past to justify claims that estrogen therapy with Premarin reduces the risk of heart attacks. However, thanks to the various studies, we now know that this is not true.

The explanation lies in the fact that triglyceride (blood fat) values increase with the use of Premarin, and this increase is associated with greater cardiovascular disease risk (see page 37).

Dr M Colgan, in his book entitled *Hormonal Health*[76], describes how he designed a computer programme that enabled him to predict the lowest Premarin estrogen levels that were still effective in raising HDL levels. He discovered that 0,33 mg of Premarin daily was as effective if not more effective than 1,25 mg in raising HDL levels without also raising blood fat levels. The usual Premarin doses are 0,65 and 1,25 mg daily.

The object of Dr Colgan's study was to find the dose of Premarin that has the lowest cancer risk, while at the same time not raising the levels of blood fats.

The table overleaf summarises the results of his studies:

CANCER RISK	PREMARIN DOSAGE(MG)	DURATION (YEARS)
75% increase	1,25	10
20% increase	1,25	immediate
0% increase	0,3	12,5

This is a remarkable result. Considered together with effects on blood fats of varying Premarin doses, these results show that a dose of 0,3 mg of Premarin does not increase cancer risk while at the same time retaining the favourable effects on blood fats associated with low-dose Premarin.

These figures represent average figures, thus the individual 'safe' dosage range may vary from 0,3–0,6 mg. The only way in which to determine the safe but effective dose in an individual is to experiment with increasing doses – starting with 0,1 mg and increasing the dose by 0,1 mg every 14 days. Maintain a 'symptoms diary', carefully noting how you feel, evidence of swollen breasts, etc; your doctor will follow changes in blood fat patterns. No woman should take more than 0,6 mg of Premarin per day for long periods (more than five years).

The above procedure is tedious, time consuming and often inaccurate, and should only be resorted to by those who insist on using Premarin.

WHY ARE CONJUGATED HORSE ESTROGENS TOXIC?

During the last few years it has become increasingly clear that certain derivatives of estrone and estradiol are sources of carcinogens that lead to breast, ovarian, endometrium and prostate cancers.

Estradiol and estrone can both be converted by oxidation into 4- and 16-hydroxy derivatives, both of which are carcinogenic, while the corresponding 2-hydroxy derivatives are non-carcinogenic and protective against cancer. (It is interesting to note that the compound indole-3-carbinol, present in broccoli and other plants of the cabbage family, shifts these conversions away from the harmful 4 and 16 derivatives toward the protective 2 derivatives). In turn, estradiol itself is converted into estrone by means of oxidation.

This does not happen in the case of estriol. The latter is also formed by further oxidation of estrone and it therefore represents an end-oxidative product (that is, it cannot be further oxidised) of the estrogens. This means that it cannot be converted into the dangerous hydroxylated derivatives. Because these by-products are formed through a process of oxidation, these reactions are likely to be suppressed in the presence of antioxidants[77].

Patients on estrogen therapy involving estradiol and Premarin (one of its constituents in estrone) should, in addition to the low doses suggested above, take additional safety precautions by also taking high levels of antioxidants such as vitamin C (1 000–2 000 mg) and vitamin E (100 mg).

At least 30% of women will not fill a prescription for horse-estrogen-based HRT, and of those who do, the majority will discontinue soon after starting because of the unpleasant side effects, which include mood changes, breast tenderness, bloating, weight gain (due to overdosage) and fear of breast cancer[78].

THE STEROID HORMONES: HOW DO THEY WORK?

The enormity of the problem of using a mixture (such as Premarin) of at least 20 estrogenic compounds (most of which do not even occur in humans) in a human being becomes clear when you consider how the steroid hormones act in the body.

The cells that respond to estrogens (there are more than 50 such types of tissue) have specific intra- and extracellular receptors with a high affinity for the particular hormone. The primary action of such a hormone, once it is inside the cell, is to bind to a particular receptor to form a hormone-receptor complex, the further actions of which determine the ultimate cellular response. This complex binds with hormone responsive regions of the genes, which ultimately elicit a particular cellular response.

Clearly each type of estrogen will have a different type of response, depending on the genes activated. Non bio-identical hormones, such as horse estrogens, act in the same way as toxins in the genes, eliciting all sorts of abnormal responses[79].

Each foreign compound may activate part of the gene complex. In that sense, the large number of non-human hormones in the CEE are comparable as a group to all other patent medicines which cause side effects because the body has never before been exposed to these compounds.

Moreover, experience has shown that the longer the period you ingest such unnatural compounds, the more likely it is that you will encounter unwanted side effects. In the case of CEE and synthetic progestogens, these side effects, unfortunately, include cancer.

BIO-IDENTICAL HORMONES AND SYNERGISTIC ACTION

The relevant bio-identical hormones are estradiol, estrone and estriol, although excessive quantities of estradiol or estrone on their own may still not be without danger.

The best approximation of a 'safe' hormone supplement is one that is able to supply the principal estrogens in the same proportion as that in which they are present in the blood.

This was first appreciated by US-based Dr Jonathan Wright, who formulated the product Triple Estrogen (sold in Europe under the name Tri-Est). It is made from hormone precursors in plants, and at the time of writing is available in South Africa under the name Tri-E. It comprises 80% estriol, 10% estradiol and 10% estrone.

No product, even if natural, is completely safe, and still has to be used under medical supervision and with careful consideration of each patient's particular circumstances. It is also desirable to monitor blood levels of the various hormones.

The benefits of estrogen supplementation, particularly with bio-identical hormones, are considerable, which is the reason why so many women insist on some form of HRT. These benefits include increased smoothness of the skin, firmness and elasticity, improved moistness of mucous membranes, including the vaginal mucosae, increased muscle tone and sex drive, less osteoporosis at least in the short term, and an increased sense of wellbeing.

MINIMISING THE SIDE EFFECTS OF HORSE ESTROGENS

One particularly nasty side effect of horse estrogen supplements is the tendency to increase blood clots (thus increasing the risk of strokes and heart attacks). Bio-identical estrogens are less inclined to do so, but there is still a risk, depending on dosage.

The best way to prevent such blood clots from forming is to take a daily supplement of omega-3 fatty acids and vitamin E (400 IU). The cheapest source of omega-3 fatty acids is the time-honoured cod-liver oil! It does not taste good but has the additional advantage of also providing important quantities of vitamin A and vitamin D.

Bio-identical estrogens have a slightly elevated cancer risk because they may also be oxidised to the carcinogenic hydroxy derivatives, but the risk is much lower than with horse estrogens. The cancer risk can be minimised by taking the lowest possible dose compatible with symptom reduction (hot flushes, depression, sleeplessness, irritability and other menopausal symptoms) and by ensuring an adequate intake of antioxidants.

In addition to these precautions and medically supervised blood level determinations, a new and sensitive test has become available which can virtually exclude the risk. It is known as the 2/16a test and measures the ratio of the harmless 2-hydroxy estrogen derivatives and the carcinogenic 16-hydroxy derivatives in the blood.

If this ratio is abnormal (it may be abnormal even in the absence of estrogen supplements), take an indole-3-carbinol (I3C) supplement, which can help shift the balance of the 2-hydroxy to 16-hydroxy estrogen derivatives to a more favourable ratio. I3C occurs in Brussels sprouts, broccoli, cabbage and cauliflower. Other supplements that may reduce the cancer risk are selenium, folic acid and omega-3 oils.

WHAT ARE THE ALTERNATIVES TO CONVENTIONAL HRT?

ESTRIOL

In addition to bio-identical hormones such as Tri-E or Tri-Est, estriol certainly deserves serious consideration.

Estriol is an end product of estrogen metabolism in humans, and is produced in large quantities during pregnancy, presumably to protect the fetus. It does not cause wild growth of cells like estradiol and estrone, and it does not cause cancer[80] – instead, it reduces the binding of carcinogenic estrogens (estradiol, estrone) to cells where they may cause cancer. A large trial in Germany showed that 2–8 mg of estriol eliminated menopausal symptoms and prevented vaginal atrophy[80].

In order to produce a bio-identical product it is best to combine estriol with small quantities of estradiol and estrone, as in the case of Tri-Est or Tri-E, which contain (per daily dose): 2,0 mg of estriol, 0,25 mg of estradiol and 0,25 mg of estrone.

The usual long-term dose of this product is 2,0 mg daily, or even less. For severe menopausal symptoms, the dose may have to be doubled temporarily.

PHYTOESTROGENS

These are plant estrogens that have been used successfully in humans for the treatment of menopausal symptoms. Although they are weak estrogens that may not work in all patients, in the majority of cases they are effective and have no serious side effects (long-term use may cause mild suppression of the thyroid gland). The most important of these estrogens are soya isoflavones; Black Cohosh; Licorice extracts; Dong Quai; and Chasteberry. Each of these have particular advantages that may be useful in a particular situation.

Black Cohosh has been shown in several clinical trials to be particularly useful for the treatment of menopausal symptoms. It is being used by more that two million women in Europe and according to one clinical study published in 1988, it was as effective as estrogens but with fewer side effects[81]. In another study, Black Cohosh produced clear improvement in menopausal symptoms in over 80% of patients in 6–8 weeks. Both physical and psychological problems improved.

THE WAY FORWARD

Do not attempt to treat your menopausal problems without proper medical guidance. Find a progressive doctor or gynaecologist who understands the importance of natural products in the treatment of disease and, above all, find one who is fully informed on the latest developments regarding HRT.

Do not use Premarin or any other preparation that contains CEE or a synthetic progestogen; that said, if you insist on using Premarin or a combined form of Premarin, do not use more than 0,6 mg per day, and do not use it for longer than four years, even with regular medical checks.

As the first option, consider estriol or the bio-identical products Tri-E or Tri-Est, and use the lowest possible dose that is effective in your case.

Do not neglect to include natural progesterone cream in your treatment programme to prevent estrogen dominance. After menopause, both estrogen and progesterone levels may be critically low due to failing ovarian production of the hormones. When only estrogen is then replaced by means of ERT, a distorted balance develops. This condition is associated with face puffiness, uterine bleeding, night swelling of feet and PMS-type symptoms.

In consultation with your doctor, do regular blood analyses to monitor your progress, even if you use a bio-identical formulation.

Do not use any form of HRT in order to prevent a heart attack or osteoporosis. When hormone replacement therapy is necessary to control menopausal symptoms, use low-dose bio-identical hormones or a plant estrogen source. This is the safest, least invasive and most gentle strategy. Best results are obtained when these are combined with conventional measures to reduce heart attacks, breast cancer and osteoporosis.

CHAPTER FOUR

HIDDEN ANAEMIA
AND EXCESSIVE IRON
SUPPLEMENTATION

At first the concepts of hidden anaemia and excessive iron supplementation seem contradictory. There are dangers associated with untreated anaemia (some of it partly due to iron deficiency), yet there are also dangers associated with too much iron.

The truth is that millions of people all over the world are needlessly dying as a result of these two situations.

Anaemia is a condition where the blood contains too few red blood cells. The condition may have a variety of causes, and iron deficiency is only one of them. Anaemia may be detected by several laboratory methods, including blood iron levels, the haematocrit value and blood ferritin.

HIDDEN ANAEMIA

Anaemia is never 'normal' – common, yes, particularly among the elderly, but this does not make it normal.

If you neglect to detect and treat anaemia, don't be too surprised if you suffer from the long-term consequences of subclinical anaemia (the stage before symptoms are noticed). However, even people who do go for checkups also appear to suffer from some degree of anaemia. Studies have shown that 24–40% of hospitalised patients over the age of 65 suffer from varying degrees of anaemia. One of the reasons is that doctors seldom consider subclinical anaemia in the elderly as important[123]. However, there is evidence to show that relatively anaemicic patients have an increased risk of heart failure, stroke and cancer, as well as an increased risk of dying from these diseases[124].

The reason for this is not difficult to understand. Anaemia is an indicator of the blood's oxygen-carrying capacity, and in the case of the elderly, where blood supply to the heart and brain may be compromised as a result of narrowing of blood vessels, the delivery of oxygen may reach dangerously lowered levels.

The importance of adequate oxygen delivery to tissues and adequate blood haemoglobin levels cannot be overemphasised. This does not apply only to the elderly, although here tissue oxygen delivery may be compromised as a result of reduced tissue perfusion. Young people, particularly athletes, also exhibit the effects of reduced haemoglobin levels. A mere 10% drop in blood haemoglobin levels severely reduces athletic performance by 20–25%[125].

In addition, there is a relationship between tissue oxygenation and cancer risk. Cancer cells, unlike normal cells, are able to use alternative energy-producing pathways by means of which the cells produce energy from fuel (carbohydrates, fats) in the absence of oxygen. This gives cancer cells an unequal advantage over normal cells under conditions of oxygen deprivation, as may occur in elderly people, with reduced oxygen delivery to tissues due to impaired blood flow through narrowed blood vessels.

Cancer cells therefore thrive in a low oxygen environment. Even borderline anaemia creates these low oxygen conditions, and therefore results in higher mortality. This is one of the reasons why cancer incidence is higher in elderly people than in younger people. (If carcinogens in the environment alone were responsible for the level of cancer prevalence in the population, you would not expect such a clearly defined age barrier).

The neglect of medical practitioners to react to blood tests that reveal anaemia or subclinical anaemia is the cause of many unnecessary and premature deaths.

EVALUATING THE ANAEMIA PATIENT

A battery of tests is available to evaluate the patient with suspected anaemia. The most important ones are: red blood cell count; serum iron; concentration; serum total iron binding capacity; serum transferrin saturation (iron stores); haemoglobin concentration; and haematocrit.

Haemoglobin is the iron-containing red blood pigment, and is responsible for the red colour of blood and red blood cells. The haematocrit is the proportion of whole blood occupied by the red blood cells, thus a haematocrit value of 43% means that 43% of the blood volume is taken up by the red blood cells. Normal values lie between 36–50%, while a reading below 36% indicates anaemia.

Since only slight deviations from normality may already be significant, it is important for you and your doctor to determine the underlying causes and to take immediate action to rectify these.

CAUSES OF ANAEMIA

Anaemia may have a number of causes other than iron deficiency, including infections (such as malaria) that destroy red blood cells, cancer and serious intestinal bleeding (such as from a bleeding ulcer).

Iron deficiency can be readily diagnosed and can be corrected by means of the right supplements, but iron alone will not correct iron-deficiency anaemia. Other important nutrients are also required for the formation of haemoglobin, such as[126] folic acid, vitamin B12, vitamin B6, zinc and copper, and vitamins C and E.

The ageing process itself may be responsible for anaemia, as people tend to become more anaemic as they age. This may be due to hormonal imbalances, because as we age, melatonin levels decline sharply, and low melatonin levels have been linked to anaemia[127]. Sublingual tablets (3 mg) are usually given to correct melatonin deficiencies.

Low levels of folic acid and vitamin B12 may also be the cause of anaemia[128], while pernicious anaemia occurs in chronic B12 deficiency.

Elevated levels of pro-inflammatory cytokines (cellular messengers) can also cause anaemia by attacking the blood cell forming proteins. Supplements that can suppress these cytokines include DHA from fish oil, vitamin K, DHEA and nettle leaf extract[129].

If supplementation with iron, melatonin, folic acid, B12 and fish oil fail to correct the anaemia, a blood analysis of hormone levels should be conducted.

Testosterone levels are frequently low in elderly men and may also be a cause of anaemia. These low levels are often due to the conversion of testosterone into estrogen, which may be harmful in several ways in addition to the accompanying anaemia. In such cases the pharmacological conversion of the administered estrogen prevents the therapy from being successful.

In elderly men, the age-associated rise in the levels of the enzyme aromatase is responsible for the increased conversion of testosterone into estrogen, with all the harmful consequences.

ANAEMIA AND HEART ATTACK

A study published in the *New England Journal of Medicine* in 2001 investigated the relationship between anaemia and mortality in elderly heart attack patients in a hospital[130].

In this study, haematocrit values were used as an indicator of anaemia. The following results were obtained.

HAEMATOCRIT %	ODDS OF DYING WITHIN 30 DAYS
5–24%	78%
24,1%–27%	52%
27,1–30%	40%
30,1–33%	31%
Above 33%	0%

These figures show that the risk of dying increases sharply when the haematocrit value is below 33%, and reaches astonishingly high values in cases of severe anaemia. Nearly eight out of ten severely anaemic patients will die within 30 days, so clearly no elderly heart patient can afford to be anaemic. The same team of doctors continued to do the next logical thing: give these anaemic patients blood transfusions and then see whether their chances of survival improved. They reported the following results:

HAEMATOCRIT VALUE	REDUCTION IN MORTALITY AFTER BLOOD TRANSFUSION
Below 24%	64%
24,1–27%	31%
27,1–30%	25%

The magnitude of the response to a blood transfusion is surprisingly large: giving a blood transfusion to such patients saved the lives of one in four people. The doctors involved in the study concluded that 'the more aggressive use of transfusions in the management of lower haematocrit levels in elderly patients with acute coronary disease may be warranted'[129].

ANAEMIA AND CANCER

Cancer cells flourish in an oxygen-poor environment[45] because they have developed the capacity to extract energy from fuels (fats and carbohydrates) in the absence of oxygen. Thus the higher the haematocrit values, the more normal cells will be advantaged relative to cancer cells, and vice versa. The situation is aggravated in the clinical management of cancer, since conventional treatments often induce anaemia, as they adversely affect the biosynthesis of haemoglobin.

The elevated levels of cytokines in someone with cancer also induce anaemia by suppressing red blood cell formation. Clinical management must include the regular determination of haematocrit values. The objective must be to ensure that the haematocrit value, red blood cell and haemoglobin values are in the upper third range of normal. The most seriously ill cancer patients are also those with the lowest haematocrit values.

Fortunately the results of one study on the effects of anaemia on the survival rates of cancer patients are available[131]. This study found that people who had anaemia and cancer had an increased mortality risk of 65%. Mild anaemia also posed an increased risk.

In South Africa oncologists seldom adequately treat anaemia in their patients, perhaps because they do not consider it important, but also because of the costs of drugs.

ANAEMIA AND THE ELDERLY

Life expectancy is not only adversely affected in elderly heart patients, but in elderly people in general. A recent study investigated the risk of dying during the next five years in anaemic elderly individuals in various age groups compared to a similar group of non-anaemic elderly patients[132]. The following results were obtained:

AGE GROUP	INCREASED RISK OF DYING COMPARED TO NON-ANAEMIC INDIVIDUALS
70–79	28%
80–89	34%
90–99	48%

Clearly anaemia is a strong indicator of early death in the elderly, regardless of whether they have heart disease or not. However, the risk is greater in the case of heart patients.

Interestingly, stroke was the cause of death most associated with anaemia, indicating the sensitivity of brain tissue to the adverse effects of tissue oxygen deprivation.

It is clear, then, that while anaemia is always undesirable, if you are over 60 it is matter of life and premature death.

THE ROLE OF IRON AND ANAEMIA

Iron in its reduced form is an essential constituent of the haemoglobin molecule. However, treating anaemia does not mean giving excessive amounts of iron. Not only does anaemia have causes unrelated to iron status, but oversupplementing with iron can have life-threatening consequences.

IRON SUPPLEMENTATION IN INFANTS

Most living organisms, with the exception of lactic acid bacteria, require the presence of iron in order to grow. When a human baby is born, its gastro-intestinal tract is sterile. Neither bacteria nor iron are present. Since lactic acid bacteria do not need iron for growth, they are the only bacteria that can grow in the baby's gastro-intestinal tract, and they start doing so after birth.

The presence of lactic acid bacteria at this stage is necessary, as it is required for the digestion of mother's milk. At this stage, the baby's immune system is poorly developed, and it relies on the antibodies derived from the mother.

The absence of iron in the gut prevents the growth of other harmful bacteria which, unlike the lactic acid bacteria, cannot grow in the absence of iron. This situation persists for as long as the baby is on mother's milk, which also contains very little iron[133]. The presence of iron in mother's milk is not necessary, because a human baby is born with a reserve iron supply of 75 mg per kilogram body weight (considerably more than in adults). This level of iron is enough to sustain at least a year's healthy growth in the infant.

The practice of using iron-enriched milk substitutes has many adverse effects on the infant, and is possibly behind the diarrhoea problems that frequently develop in infants on milk formulae. Even though iron is needed for the manufacture of haemoglobin in the red blood cells, the infant carries adequate supplies of iron and does not need such an external supply of iron.

Iron supplements given unnecessarily and in excess are harmful for everyone, but in the case of infants, the effects are dramatic and readily visible.

It is astonishing, then, that the RDA (Recommended Daily Allowances) values in both the United States and South Africa have entries for iron supplements in the zero to one-year age group!

IRON SUPPLEMENTATION IN LATER LIFE

Large quantities of iron tablets are still prescribed indiscriminately and unnecessarily. Since excess iron stimulates free radical formation, and since free radicals are linked to many diseases, it is easy to see why widespread and unnecessary supplementation with iron can be linked to many diseases.

In 1975 Professor Weinberg of the University of Indiana published research that showed how iron fortification of foods (such as 50 mg per kg of flour) resulted in the increased incidence of disease[134], particularly infections.

Universal fortification of iron is therefore wrong, as there are many areas where people do in fact get enough iron from food. A total intake (food plus supplements) of more than 20 mg of iron a day can be considered excessive[135].

Yet iron is still the most widely prescribed nutrient.

HOW COMMON IS IRON DEFICIENCY?

A study published in the *Journal of the American Medical Association* in 1997 showed that children and premenstrual women are most likely to suffer from iron deficiency[140]. South African figures are likely to be similar.

In these groups iron deficiency is a real problem and supplementation is indicated.

POPULATION GROUP	% WITH IRON DEFICIENCY	WITH IRON DEFICIENCY ANAEMIA	ACTUAL NUMBER
Children (1–2 years)	9	3	700 000
Premenopausal women	9–11	2–5	7 800 000

However, most men and the vast majority of women are not deficient, and do not need supplements. To extrapolate the needs of such a small group to everybody and therefore to supplement universally (in food-enrichment schemes) is unwise and could even be hazardous.

Iron should be given strictly only to those who need it, and should not be included in any multinutrient supplement intended for long-term use by everyone. Nor should it be included in fortified foods intended for general consumption – those companies that still include iron as one of the ingredients of a multinutrient formula probably are not aware of the latest research.

HOW MUCH IRON?

In the case of all other groups other than menstruating women, the body is virtually a closed tank as far as iron is concerned. In contrast to most other minerals, iron is not lost in the urine, and daily losses are limited to the small amounts in cells lost daily in the gastro-intestinal tract and skin. This amounts to 1,0 mg/day.

In the case of athletes, additional losses occur as a result of sweating and hemolysis (red blood cell breakage resulting from sudden pressures arising when the feet strike the ground, such as in marathon running or when muscles are contracted).

In order to determine total daily requirements for purposes of supplementation, it is best to consider the total daily loss of iron in different groups of people, such as menstruating and non-menstruating women, men and children. Taking into account that only 10% of administered iron is absorbed, research shows that men and non-menstruating women need 10 mg of iron, menstruating women 15 mg, pregnant women 25 mg and male blood donors 30 mg.

Iron absorption from the diet is normally about 10 mg per day. This shows that men and non-menstruating women do not need any supplemental iron. Menstruating women need about 5–10 mg while pregnant women need 15–20 mg and male blood donors 20 mg per day. Doctors should never prescribe more than that.

In the case of people with a clearly established iron-deficiency-anaemia that do not respond to supplementation at these levels, the problem lies not in the dose but elsewhere. Usually the problem lies in a deficiency of the synergistic vitamins and minerals required for blood formation, such as zinc, copper, vitamin B12 and folic acid.

CHAPTER FIVE

HIV AND AIDS:
ANOTHER
PERSPECTIVE

According to current estimates, one billion people will be infected by the human immunodeficiency virus (HIV), and will develop Acquired Immune Deficiency Syndrome (AIDS) by 2015, a mere 11 years from now. By that time, at least 250 million people will have died of AIDS. The vast majority (more than 80%) of these cases will be in sub-Saharan Africa.

There is little reason to believe that the epidemic will subside in the foreseeable future, or that some effective form of treatment will be developed. Neither antiretroviral drugs nor vaccines have much long-term success because of the extreme variability of the virus (its capacity to adapt) and because the virus hides inside immune cells where it is inaccessible to both drugs and vaccines.

What is more important is to investigate the possibilities of preventing the disease, and carefully examine the environmental circumstances in those countries where the incidence of the disease is unexpectedly low.

WHAT IS HIV?

HIV is a retrovirus, meaning that its genetic code is 'written' in RNA 'language' (a type of nucleic acid), while the genetic code of the host is written in DNA 'language'. The virus uses the host's genetic material for its own replication, but before it can do so, it has to convert its own code from RNA into DNA 'language' during the process of transcription. After infection, the virus appears in the blood and the person becomes HIV positive. The virus then starts to replicate (at different rates in different people), attacking the cells of the immune system.

When the CD4 (T-helper immune cell) count drops to below 200/mcl, clinical symptoms such as pneumonia, and increased susceptibility to opportunistic infections, start to appear. When these symptoms appear, the person is considered to have AIDS.

WHAT MAKES HIV SO DIFFICULT TO TREAT?

It is not easy to make a vaccine for one type of HI virus, as there is no such thing, strictly speaking. HIV is extremely variable, because as it transcribes itself from its own RNA coded system to a DNA code (to make it compatible with the host cells), it undergoes genetic errors. Many such errors can occur during this replication process, and the result can be a large number of viruses not quite identical to the original virus[152].

Some of these variants may be resistant to antiretrovirals (ARVs) and even vaccines developed against the original strain, which is why treatment usually involves a number of different drugs or combinations. Even when such drug combinations are used, the virus may still hide in the immune cells only to reappear later in an altered and difficult-to-treat form.

Furthermore, the infecting viruses may 'hide' by penetrating the cell membranes in certain cells, making them inaccessible to drugs and vaccines. Thus within days of initial infection, HIV may enter 'resting' T-cells of the immune system[153].

These cells are very good places to hide because they are not actively involved in the immune response and therefore escape detection by the immune system or exposure to drugs. (Before a drug can be effective, some form of activity, such as virus and/or cell multiplication, must take place.) Such resting T-cells are able to exist in a resting state for many years without showing any activity, thus offering ideal hiding places for the virus.

GETTING TO THE ROOT OF THE CAUSE

In the past, people were able to overcome major disasters only after coming to a clear understanding of the cause. Today, although many medical people believe that the cause of AIDS is clear, there are others who believe that there is, in fact, no clear understanding of the cause of AIDS, nor is there a reasonable chance that such an understanding will be forthcoming in the near future.

No real progress will be possible until an issue that has been plaguing human beings for more than 100 years is finally resolved: should treatment be directed at the external causes of diseases (micro-organisms in the case of infections, cholesterol in the case of heart disease, cancerous growths in the case of cancer), or should treatment be directed at strengthening the body's own defence mechanisms.

To this day, the bulk of medical research is aimed at developing a magic bullet or super drug, despite warnings by medical scientists such as Louis Pasteur that 'the host is more important than the invader'.

Now HIV and AIDS has appeared and the scene is set for a repeat performance of failed drug treatment. When it became known that HIV was present in the blood of people with AIDS, the medical profession adopted the standard approach: kill the invader! Accordingly, drugs such as AZT, DDC and 3TC were developed that not only killed the virus in laboratory experiments but also actually led to the temporary improvement of people living with HIV.

In turn, this encouraged the investment of many more millions of dollars in the development of yet more drugs. But still the AIDS pandemic continues, because drug treatment, while offering temporary relief to some, has not offered any real solution to the problem.

One of the assumptions about HIV/AIDS is that it is simply a virus-mediated infection and that a person will develop AIDS if he or she is infected. But why is there such an enormous difference between the infection rates (and progression to AIDS) in some closely related countries such as Senegal and the Ivory Coast or Zimbabwe? Is it because AIDS is caused only as a result of infection with the virus, or are some other factors involved?

The history of the disease supports the idea that at least one of its causes is an infectious virus. In some areas of the USA, for example, most cases occurred in drug users, many of whom shared contaminated needles. The pattern in which the disease spread from an initial focus of infection is that of an ever-expanding circle focused on the original epicentre[154], a pattern typical of infections.

On the other hand, though, there is a small group of researchers headed by Dr P Duesberg that believes HIV is merely a harmless passenger virus, and that AIDS is the end stage of the destruction of the immune system. (Dr Duesberg is a California-based microbiologist and former consultant to the South African government, known for his opposition to current medical thinking about AIDS.)

This destruction could be the result of the long-term cumulative effect of drugs (recreational and pharmaceutical), including some of the ARVs such as AZT, as well as the many other chemicals to which we are regularly exposed.

However, one of the arguments that can be used against the Duesberg theory is the fact that in sub-Saharan Africa, there has been no long-term use of drugs; nor has the developing world been as exposed to chemicals as the developed world.

Most people believe that AIDS is caused by HIV alone, and this view was widely supported by doctors and researchers from around the world who attended the International AIDS Conference in Durban in July 2000. This view was formally enshrined in the 'Durban Declaration'[155], issued after the conference. In this document, the vast majority (5 018) of those attending the conference stated that 'HIV is the sole cause of AIDS'.

This confirms the widely held medical point of view and stresses the necessity of finding a drug that will kill the virus itself. By implication, if such a drug could be found, the problem would be solved. Obviously such a line of thinking suits the pharmaceutical industry. In scientific disputes of this nature, though, the majority point of view has often been wrong.

Clearly the truth cannot be determined by vote. And in the case of the Durban Declaration, politics and financial interests also played a role: the current South African president, a politician with no scientific training, also became involved in the dispute, both before and after the conference.

EVIDENCE IN SUPPORT OF THE DURBAN DECLARATION

All people living with AIDS are carriers of HIV, most of whom will show signs of opportunistic infections 5–10 years from the time of infection.

The number of AIDS-defining clinical conditions normally used in the diagnosis of the disease include: tuberculosis, pneumocystis carinii pneumonia (known as PCP, a rare pneumonia attacking only people with weak immune systems), histoplasmosis, cryptococcal and TB meningitis, toxoplasmosis (causing a stroke), cytomegalovirus (also known as CMV, the gradual deterioration of eyesight), herpes simplex infections, mycobacterial infections and others reflecting a general reduced capacity to resist opportunistic infections. In Africa, infected patients die much sooner.

HIV-infected people can be identified by antibody detection as well as viral isolation tests generally used to identify virus infections.

People who receive HIV-infected blood or blood products will develop the disease, while those treated with uninfected blood will not.

Up to 20% of children born to HIV-positive mothers will also develop the disease, and the chances of such a transmission occurring increases with the viral load in the mother.

In laboratory tests, HIV has been shown to specifically attack the T-helper (CD4) cells of the immune system. However, the percentage of CD4 cells attacked is low (in some instances less than 1%), making it difficult to explain the disease on this basis.

Drugs and drug combinations that are known to block viral replication in the laboratory have been shown to benefit people with AIDS in the short term.

Clearly the arguments above are significant and support the fact that a virus is involved, but they do not prove that other, contributory factors are not also involved.

ANOMALIES IN THE HIV DEBATE

The worrisome facts that weaken ruling theories of the day are the anomalies that ultimately lead to the revelations that bring us closer to the truth. These anomalies are named 'the termites of science' by Prof Harold D Foster in *What Really Causes AIDS*[157].

Fortunately, there is also a middle ground – between the 'virus-only' theory and the 'non-virus' theory – which appears to be much nearer to the truth.

This middle ground is occupied by a group of scientists led by Prof Foster (based at the University of British Columbia in Canada) and Dr EW Taylor (at the University of Georgia in the USA). They accept that a virus is involved, but point out that for the virus to exert its full effect, certain nutritional conditions are a prerequisite. In other words, while HIV is a necessary cause of AIDS, it is not a sufficient cause.

This middle ground pays attention to antioxidants, and the role that free radicals could play in promoting the development of clinical AIDS, while Prof Foster has revealed studies that explain many of the anomalies associated with the 'virus-only' theory.

The following is a brief summary of the principal anomalies and observations, many of them based on epidemiological surveys, which the 'virus-only' theory cannot explain, or has difficulty accounting for.

DIFFERENT COUNTRIES, DIFFERENT DISEASE INCIDENCE

It is assumed that HIV has its origins in Africa, and it is here that the spread of the disease has been most rapid. The infection is particularly rife in sub-Saharan Africa, where countries share many lifestyle and dietary practices.

The following table gives an overview of the disease prevalence in antenatal clinics in some of these countries. The table uses the most recent statistics, but although these are in some instances six years old, it is unlikely that the picture can change so dramatically in so short a time so as to alter the conclusions reached here. Each country below has the same type of HIV.

COUNTRY	INCIDENCE %	ANNUAL MORTALITY PER 1 000 000 OF POPULATION
UGANDA[158]	14 (1998) 31 (1990)	5 202
SOUTH AFRICA[159]	19	6 265
SENEGAL[160]	0,5	844

The first two entries in this table reflect the disease situation in virtually all the sub-Saharan countries. The only remarkable feature about the incidence of HIV infection and AIDS here is the alarming rate at which incidence increases and spreads[156 & 157].

The exception is Senegal where the population is among the most sexually active in African countries. Accurate information is available on the prevalence and incidence of HIV and AIDS in sex trade workers in the capital city Dakar, because the Senegalese government has been registering prostitutes since 1966 (long before the onset of the epidemic) to control other sexually transmitted diseases such as gonorrhea and syphilis[161].

Polygamy is common and legally sanctioned in Senegal, where men may have up to four wives. In addition, promiscuity is high, even among married men. When a married man searches for additional wives, he almost invariably 'samples' many others before making a decision[162].

A survey conducted in 1997 found that 33% of Senegalese males aged 15–49 years admitted to recently having sex with other partners, and a large percentage of these were not using condoms[163].

These data show that Senegal is a country where the level of sexual activity is very high, including a high level of unprotected sex with non-regular partners.

On the basis of this, you would expect that the incidence of HIV and AIDS would be high and that the disease would be spreading rapidly.

As the table shows, and as commented on by some researchers[157], the opposite appears to be true. Not only is the incidence of the disease 10–20 times lower than in most other countries in the region, but the rate of dissemination appears to be very low, if indeed it is spreading at all. What is it about the environment in Senegal that dissuades the virus from proliferating?

It would appear that Senegal has an ideal environment for the support of the immune system, as a result of which the incidence of cancer[179] and AIDS[160] is extremely low.

Senegal is rich in phosphorite, a mineral deposit containing calcium phosphate, which is extremely rich in selenium; it is now mined for its phosphate content[180]. The nutritional environment in Senegal is largely determined by these minerals, which are also rich in calcium and magnesium.

Only a small percentage of the annual rainfall in Senegal runs off into its rivers – the rest is retained in the soil. People are therefore largely dependent on ground water, which is in contact with the selenium and mineral-rich soil deposits. The result is that the drinking water in Senegal has the highest calcium and magnesium salt content in the world[181], and very low levels of toxic heavy minerals such as mercury, presumably due in part to the absence of heavy industries.

In contrast, in those African countries where HIV infection is high and it progresses rapidly toward clinical AIDS, the soil selenium levels are invariably low[182].

Within our immune systems, there are two main groups of immune cells, the B-lymphocytes (which produce antibodies) and the T-lymphocytes which attack invaders directly (see chapter 7 for more information regarding the immune system).

The T-cells are subdivided into T-helper cells (CD4) and T-suppressor cells (CD8), each with specific functions in maintaining overall immunity. These different types of immune cells must remain in balance. The T-helper cells are also called CD4 cells.

These lymphocytes play an extremely important role in maintaining immune function by signalling other immune cells to carry out their specific functions, so as to ensue a co-ordinated immune response to any external threat.

One of the consequences of HIV infection is that the number of CD4 cells declines, thus disturbing the balance between the CD4 and the CD8 cells. In a healthy person, the number of CD4 cells is 800–1 200/mcl of blood.

If the CD4 cell count falls below 200/mcl, the person becomes increasingly vulnerable to opportunistic infections, frequently seen in people with AIDS. Generally, the CD4 count is used as a guide of immune function in people with HIV or AIDS.

Interestingly, though, the CD4 count is not the most reliable indicator of survival. According to Prof Foster, the concentration of selenium in the blood plasma is a far more reliable indicator of whether HIV will become AIDS[167]. In other words, life expectancy is indicated not by CD4 count but by the amount of selenium in the body.

MATERNAL MORTALITY PATTERNS

The rate of HIV transmission by breast-feeding varies from 14% to 26%, depending on the timing of maternal infection, the viral load and, presumably, the selenium status of mother and infant. The fact that the virus may be transmitted in the mother's milk comes as no surprise, and is consistent with the theory that the disease is caused at least partly by a virus. However, the finding that the transmission rate is so low (one in every five babies fed on the milk of HIV-positive mothers) is rather surprising.

A Kenyan study published in the *Lancet* in 2001 shows that breast-feeding is associated with an increased mortality rate in nursing mothers[165].

This is indeed unexpected, at least in terms of the popular 'virus-only' theory, because the nursing of a baby does not affect the virus level in the mother, but it does cause the loss of selenium.

In this study the sum total of all the women who died in the breast-feeding group within two years was three times higher than in a formula-fed control group.

Breast-feeding by an HIV-positive mother thus seems to reduce her life expectancy and increases the likelihood that she will succumb as a result of the disease. It also reduces the life expectancy of the baby who is being breast-fed. This study clearly indicates that breast-feeding has a negative impact on the mother's immune system.

The fact that the breast-feeding mother's life is shortened as a result of breast-feeding cannot be explained by the 'virus-only' theory; it can be explained, though, by the important role of selenium in the development of AIDS. In order to develop clinical AIDS, the mother must be selenium deficient, and because the mother is deficient, her baby will also be deficient. Hence the risk is increased for mother and child, but because of the loss of selenium in her milk to the baby, the already-deficient mother's risk will be increased.

KAPOSI'S SARCOMA

Kaposi's sarcoma is a cancer that was rarely seen before 1980, but today it is recognised as the most common form of cancer in people with HIV – to the extent that it is considered a marker for the disease.

Kaposi's sarcoma mainly affects the skin (purplish spots), although other organs of the body may also be infected.

Kaposi's sarcoma was first described by Moritz Kaposi in 1872, but since the 1950s it began to regularly appear in patients in Kenya and other equatorial African countries. Early in the 1980s, when AIDS first came to the attention of the medical world, it also began to appear regularly among the gay population in the New York area.

Subsequent research revealed that the lesions in Kaposi's sarcoma (also known as Kaposi's tumour) contained a new type of virus, the human herpes virus 8 (HHV8) or Kaposi-associated virus (KSHV)[166]. This virus is closely linked to HIV infection[167]. While the cancer can occur in the absence of HIV, it rarely does, hence the low incidence of Kaposi's tumour prior to the appearance of HIV. On the other hand, AIDS can and does develop in many patients without evidence of Kaposi's sarcoma. Thus some sort of symbiotic relationship appears to occur between the two viruses. Prof Foster suggests that both viruses require the [168] same nutritional cofactors such as selenium in order to become virulent[155].

WHY NOW?

There is evidence that humans are not the natural hosts of HIV. There are at least 26 different strains of a similar virus in apes, and these may cause simian immuno-deficiency disease (SIV). Two of these simian viruses have mutated to give rise to HIV1 and HIV2 in humans. These viruses have evolved from simian viruses that have entered the human population by cross-species transmission.

In West Central Africa, monkeys and chimpanzees are hunted for the 'bush meat' trade, and are subsequently eaten by humans. The conditions under which butchers slaughter these animals are very unhygienic indeed[169]. The 'bush meat' trade has been flourishing for a long time, possibly for centuries, which has offered any number of opportunities for such cross-species exchange of viruses to occur. Moreover, there was ample opportunity for the HIV1 and HIV2 viruses to spread to the Western world during the widespread slave trade.

Why, then, did the AIDS epidemic begin only about 20 years ago?

The answer given by Prof Foster is that cross-species transmission of simian viruses to humans has occurred countless times but when it did, development of the human equivalents of these viruses did not occur since they lacked the cofactors or other circumstances required for the growth of these viruses[155].

However, such factors have been introduced into the environment only recently. The development of nutritional deficiencies offers the most reasonable answer to this question.

THE INVASION OF IMMUNE CELLS

One of the typical attributes of HIV/AIDS is the distortion of the immune system, which is mainly manifested as a critical lowering of the number of CD4 (T-helper) cells.

It has therefore been thought that the disease results from the destruction of CD4 cells by the virus. However, the extent to which this destruction happens initially appears to be insignificant. Estimates of the infection rate of CD4 cells in the blood varies from one in 10 000 to one in 100[170].

In addition, there is evidence to show that long before the numbers of CD4 cells decline, the CD4 cells of the patient lose their ability to respond to foreign antigens [155].

NUTRIENTS, HIV AND AIDS

During the last 15 years, several thousand scientific and medical studies have shown that HIV-related immune cell destruction directly correlates with deficiencies of certain nutrients (minerals, vitamins, amino acids) and certain hormones such as DHEA[171].

These studies indicate that the use of the proper combination of nutrients, especially the antioxidants, may not only retard damage to the immune system but may also be an effective way of restoring immune competence in HIV-positive patients, especially those who are in the early stages of the disease.

In discussing the various nutrients that have been shown to play a role in HIV and AIDS (and particularly in designing treatment strategies), it is important to distinguish between two groups of nutrients.

Group 1 nutrients are those that are encoded by the virus during replication: selenium, cysteine, glutamine and tryptophan. These are increasingly being consumed as the virus replicates. They are therefore of prime importance in connection with the way in which the disease progresses, and also offer the best prospects of therapeutic intervention.

Group 2 nutrients are those that are also depleted in the process of viral replication but are not subject to the multiplication effect. Although also of great importance in the person with HIV or AIDS, these nutrients are less critical than those in the first group. Most of the nutrients in this group are powerful antioxidants.

GLUTATHIONE

One such critical nutrient is glutathione (GSH), as the HI virus severely depletes the cells of this important amino acid derivative. Glutathione is a tripeptide, consisting of three amino acids (glutamic acid, cysteine and glycine), and is produced in every cell by means of biochemical reactions.

It is always dangerous to designate one particular nutrient as being more important than others, because of the important principle of nutrient synergism (the interdependence of nutrients). However, if such a designation were possible, the sulphur-containing tripeptide GSH would be a strong candidate.

GSH is present in all living cells, where it acts as a scavenger of a variety of toxins. As an antioxidant, it reacts with free radicals, including the dangerous oxygen free radicals such as superoxides and hydroxyl radicals. GSH is therefore an important protector against oxidative stress, chemical and metabolic[172] toxins and, say the latest findings, viruses.

This multifunctional control of many cellular processes elevates GSH to the status of 'controller of all living systems'; GSH also controls our living systems' capacity to adapt to changing circumstances, including their ability to repel attacks by toxins and viruses. Moreover, it is the one antioxidant that is present in nearly all cells of all organisms and, as such, it represents the cell's first line of defence against invading organisms such as viruses.

The liver is an important source of circulating GSH, although the levels of GSH decline with age. Research suggests that people who maintain high levels of GSH, for whatever reason, have extreme longevity[169]. In people with chronic diseases and infections, including HIV and AIDS, GSH levels are significantly lower than in healthy controls.

GSH has numerous other important functions in the body, some of which are directly related to HIV and AIDS. It is necessary for maintaining immune-mediated T-cell activation, and it also helps to maintain the balance between the T-helper cells 1 and 2[173].

The amount of GSH in blood plasma has been found to be depressed as early as three weeks after infection with HIV and long before symptoms of clinical AIDS appear[174]. Intracellular levels of GSH in both CD4 and CD8 cells have been found to be severely depressed (62–69% of normal values). This finding is significant in view of the finding that a reduction of 10–40% in the levels of GSH completely inhibited T-cell activation.

The depletion of cellular glutathione levels also partly explains the decrease of protein synthesis seen in people with HIV and AIDS, in the form of 'wasting'. In addition, the intestinal impairment caused by a glutathione deficiency often manifests as inflammatory bowel disease, a common problem in people with HIV/AIDS, and which prevents effective absorption of vitally needed nutrients (see chapter 7).

AIDS-associated deficiency of glutathione leads to the build-up of enormous levels of oxidative stress, which damages and kills many healthy cells in the body, including those of the immune system.

Is it possible to raise blood glutathione levels?

Several approaches to raising blood levels of glutathione are being explored. One is the administration of GSH itself, and another approach is to give orally the precursors of GSH (eg N-acetylcysteine) in order to stimulate endogenous synthesis of GSH.

Other substances that boost GSH levels are selenium (600 mcg a day); vitamin C (5 000 mg); lipoic acid (600 mg); whey protein (40 g); S-adenosylmethionine (600 mg); and N-acetylcysteine (NAC) (1 800 mg). At present, the use of the cysteine precursor NAC appears to be the most effective method.

How do HIV and AIDS affect glutathione levels?

Numerous studies have shown that HIV severely depletes cells of available GSH. These studies have also shown that the lack of GSH reduces the effectiveness of the lymphocytes by reducing the number of CD4 cells. This contributes to the immune cell impairment so characteristic of AIDS.

GSH levels predict life expectancy

The results of a randomised controlled trial designed to study the effect of GSH levels on the life expectancy of people with AIDS was published in 1997[175]. The results of the New York-based study showed that GSH levels predicted poor life expectancy for people with a CD4 count below 200 as well as a low level of GSH. These people had a 20% chance of surviving the next three years, while those with a similar CD4 count but adequate GSH levels had a 60–80% chance of surviving the next three years.

A follow-up study found that similar patients who had taken N-acetylcysteine (NAC) supplements had considerably better survival rates than people who had not been treated with NAC.

Although these studies were conducted on relatively small numbers of patients and therefore need confirmation, it may be concluded that GSH blood levels predict survival rates in people with low CD4 counts and people living with AIDS benefit from taking selenium supplements. Up to 8 000 mg of NAC daily, in divided doses, was used in some of these patients. Such a high dose was generally well tolerated. Lower doses, such as 1 000–3 000 mg, are also effective but it is advisable to take NAC supplements in combination with high doses of vitamin C (3 000–5 000 mg daily, in divided doses).

Why is glutathione so important?

Glutathione (GSH) is of pivotal importance in all cells, and without adequate levels of GSH, cells will die. One molecule of GSH is lost (consumed) for every molecule of foreign toxin or virus detoxified, and there is thus a high demand for GSH in cells. In order for this demand to be met, GSH must either be constantly formed from its constituent amino acids (eg from cysteine or NAC) or it must be regenerated.

Glutathione cellular activity can be compromised when there is either a lack of building blocks (cysteine and the cofactors that are required for GSH synthesis) or when there is a deficiency of the enzyme glutathione reductase, which is necessary for the regeneration of reduced glutathione.

Adequate levels of GSH in cells are maintained through de novo synthesis and through reduction of oxidised glutathione to GSH for which the enzyme glutathione reductase (cofactors: riboflavin, magnesium) is required. In the de novo synthesis of glutathione, intracellular cysteine is a critical requirement.

Glutathione reacts with deadly free radicals, such as peroxides and other reactive oxygen species, in a reaction catalysed by the enzyme glutathione peroxidase (cofactors: selenium, magnesium and niacin). Selenium is a critical part of this enzyme.

THE SELENIUM–HIV AND AIDS CONNECTION

This close association of the incidence and severity of HIV and AIDS with selenium levels answers many of the previously unexplained facts about the disease. This includes the fact that in infected patients, low plasma selenium levels are a better indicator of mortality risk than depressed T-lymphocyte (CD4) cell counts, which have until now been used to assess risk in patients[167].

This association between selenium and HIV and AIDS is so strong and consistent, in fact, that in the recently published *Selenium World Atlas*, the incidence of HIV is used as a surrogate measure of soil selenium levels in those countries where information on the selenium soil levels is not available[177]. This raises the question of which comes first in the person with HIV and AIDS: the low selenium levels or the low CD4 count? According to

Prof Foster, the primary event is the low selenium levels and therefore, not surprisingly, the low selenium levels are the more reliable indicator of risk, as selenium is necessary for the production of T-lymphocytes[155].

The sequence of events is therefore as follows: Low selenium leads to reduced lymphocyte production and therefore increased susceptibility to virus infections and increased opportunistic infections.

Some of these infections include viruses that are also selenium dependent, such as the Coxsackie virus (Keshan disease) and Kaposi's sarcoma (herpes virus). A possible explanation for the flourishing of these viruses in the selenium-deficient person is that the virus requires selenium to become virulent, and the reduced lymphocyte count then allows it to proliferate.

Keshan disease is an endemic human heart (cardiomyopathy) disease that is strictly limited to certain environments and geographical areas[183] and is an example of how a selenium-deficiency disease can be effectively treated with mass supplementation in whole populations.

It is a typical example of a disease where the virulence of the virus is increased in the presence of a selenium deficiency. In this case, the Coxsackie virus B3 attacks the heart muscle. The disease is limited to the so-called 'disease belt' in China (which crosses the country from northeast to southwest) and in certain areas of Korea. These different areas and zones all have one thing in common: low soil selenium content.

The Coxsackie virus (like the HI virus) encodes glutathione peroxidase and therefore depletes the host of selenium as it replicates[184]. The Chinese government has successfully implicated various strategies of increasing selenium intake in these areas, with the result that the incidence of the disease is declining[185].

The association between low selenium levels and HIV and AIDS also explains the close association between the incidence of Kaposi sarcoma and HIV and AIDS. Kaposi's sarcoma is endemic in Uganda and other selenium-deficient areas of Africa.

The basis for this competition between virus and host for selenium lies in the vital role glutathione plays in the host, as the regeneration of glutathione requires the selenium-containing enzyme glutathione peroxidase (GPx).

HIV also requires selenium because it encodes the selenium-containing GPx. This means that the virus cannot replicate without competing with its host, and in so doing, it deprives the host of vital glutathione, one of the most important cellular protectors known.

GROUP ONE NUTRIENTS

These nutrients, selenium, cysteine, glutamine and tryptophan, are consumed by the virus as it replicates. Glutathione activity levels in the body can be depleted by depressed glutathione peroxidase activity (which is necessary for glutathione to perform its biochemical function) or by a lack of the nutrients necessary for the de novo synthesis of glutathione in the body.

In the person with HIV and AIDS, this depletion results from the proliferation of HIV, which encodes not only glutathione peroxidase but also the constituent amino acids necessary for glutathione production.

Both systems have the typical features of a positive feedback system, ie, the more the virus grows, the greater the deficiencies that result from its growth. In the case of the constituent amino acids necessary for the production of glutathione, it happens because glutathione inhibits reverse transcriptase, an enzyme necessary for virus reproduction. Therefore the more the virus grows, the more it depletes the body of these vital nutrients, making it easier for the virus to replicate as serum glutathione levels decline.

Reverse transcriptase is necessary for the virus to convert its own RNA into DNA, which is required for the virus to incorporate its genetic code into the host cell genes. Therefore the removal of glutathione, the inhibitor which retards this process, will make virus replication easier.

The four basic components of glutathione peroxidase encoded by HIV are selenium, cysteine, glutamine and tryptophan. During virus replication, serious depletion of these nutrients may occur in the host[187], and this depletion is responsible for some of the major symptoms of AIDS including immune system collapse, muscle wasting, dermatitis, diarrhoea and dementia.

Foster[188] has suggested that AIDS is the clinical end-result of this process of multiple nutrient deficiencies, and that effective treatment must include supplementation with these nutrients. Supporting evidence is available from many other studies[189].

Selenium deficiency

Many of the symptoms seen in the person with AIDS can be related to a deficiency of selenium. Thus it has been suggested that declining selenium levels are directly responsible for the decline in CD4 cells, which permits the uncontrolled proliferation of opportunistic infections. Selenium (in the form of glutathione peroxidase) is essential for the production of lymphocytes.

In this theory of HIV and AIDS, selenium deficiency is seen as the primary event that leads to a decline in CD4 cells, which is in contrast to the more commonly held belief that the CD4 cell decline is caused by the destruction of these cells by the virus.

The low thyroid function seen in many people with AIDS is also due to selenium deficiency. Selenium is necessary for the conversion of T4 into T3, the biologically active form of the thyroid hormone.

Cysteine deficiency

Several studies have demonstrated the low cysteine levels in people with AIDS. Since cysteine is the controlling amino acid in the biosynthesis of glutathione, a cysteine deficiency is associated with a shortage of glutathione, with all the serious consequences this implies. Several studies have shown that supplementation with cysteine (as N-acetylcysteine) can replenish glutathione levels in CD4 cells.

Glutamine deficiency

Glutamine is an important nutrient for rapidly dividing cells such as those in the immune system and in the gut – all such cells are dependent on glutamine as their primary source of energy.

Many people with AIDS have both a glutamine deficiency and abnormal intestinal permeability associated with digestive problems and loss of protein. Supplementation with 8 g of glutamine daily can correct these. Other studies have demonstrated the value of glutamine supplements in counteracting protein loss[189], also typical of the person with AIDS.

HIV infection induces a glutamine deficiency, possibly as a result of the rapid turnover of immune cells[194]. Glutamine appears to be depleted even in asymptomatic people, but large doses (more than 20 g daily) are required to restore glutamine status to normality.

A double-blind placebo-controlled study published in 1999 demonstrated reversal of loss of lean body mass in people with AIDS when very high doses (40 g or more) of glutamine were given[195].

Remarkably, this study showed that the results in the supplemented group were similar to the lean body mass gained with recombinant growth hormone (r-hGH), currently the most effective FDA approved treatment for protein and lean body weight loss in AIDS at approximately a thirtieth of the cost. Both preparations are equally effective but the cost savings associated with the use of glutamine are substantial indeed.

Tryptophan deficiency

Tryptophan (an essential amino acid) levels in people with AIDS may be severely depressed[190], and this may be responsible for some of the symptoms seen in these patients (dementia, diarrhoea, dermatitis, death).

GROUP TWO NUTRIENTS

These are certain antioxidants that the virus does not encode but which nonetheless play an important role in controlling the infection and the metabolic consequences arising from the presence of the virus.

Antioxidants play a critical role in preventing apoptosis (programmed cell death) and viral replication in AIDS.

Lipoic acid

Lipoic acid is a versatile yet powerful antioxidant, which can protect most cell types (including cells of the immune system) against free radical attack. It has attracted much attention in HIV and AIDS research as a result of its ability to significantly raise glutathione levels in T-lymphocytes (by between 30 and 70%) both in the body and in the laboratory[191]. In addition, it interrupts virus replication directly as well as through inhibition of NF-KB (one of the factors responsible for cell death in people with AIDS), and also inhibits reverse transcriptase in a way that is synergistic with the drug AZT.

Unfortunately no large-scale clinical trials on the use of lipoic acid in people with HIV and AIDS have been published, although anecdotal experience on its use for this purpose is encouraging.

L-carnitine

Carnitine is a non-essential amino acid that transports fatty acids across cell membranes into the energy-producing mitochondria in cells.

Apoptosis, or programmed cell death, is thought to be a mechanism whereby cells, including immune cells, die off. Various studies have shown that there is a decrease in apoptosis in CD4 and CD8 cells after the addition of carnitine[196]. This has also been demonstrated in a clinical trial with asymptomatic HIV-positive patients.

The use of L-carnitine in protecting neural tissue and mitochondria against damage induced by antiviral drugs is also warranted.

Co-enzyme Q10

Q10 is important in the production of cellular energy because of its role in the electron transport chain during the liberation of energy from fuels. Q10 deficiencies have been demonstrated in people with AIDS, with the Q10 blood levels dropping as the disease progresses. However, it has also been demonstrated that supplementation has beneficial effects, with many of the typical symptoms improving after treatment with 200 mg daily of Q10[197]. Substantial increases in the CD4 and CD8 cells have also been seen after supplementation.

HORMONAL ABNORMALITIES

In the body, the hormones are produced in a step-by-step progression of chemical reactions, where cholesterol is converted into the male and female hormones. This is known as the hormonal cascade. Hormones and hormonal imbalances play a critical role in the sex lives of both men and women. In addition, they have wide-ranging metabolic effects that play an important role in regulating the immune system, and as such they are of importance to the person living with HIV and AIDS.

DHEA (DIHYDROEPIANDROSTERONE)

Several major studies have shown that HIV-infection progresses at an accelerated rate when serum levels of DHEA are low[177]. DHEA occurs in one of the steps of the hormonal cascade, and is an immediate precursor to testosterone and the estrogens. It has many other important biological functions that are unrelated to its function as a precursor of the sex hormones. For this reason, it is advisable for people with AIDS to do regular determinations of blood hormone levels (including DHEA, cortisone and TSH) and to correct these when levels are abnormal. Unfortunately, this is an expensive test, and cannot easily be considered in the treatment of whole populations.

Adequate DHEA may prevent general immune system collapse.

DHEA does not have a direct antiviral action. Its beneficial effects appear to be related to its capacity to protect the immune system against a variety of assaults.

It is probably a good idea for people living with HIV and AIDS to take a DHEA supplement, preferably under medical guidance. These are cheaper than antiretroviral drugs. The daily dose varies from 25–75 mg depending on the patient's blood level and condition. However, it is important to note that patients with liver damage must only use DHEA under medical supervision.

CORTISOL

HIV and AIDS causes a significant amount of stress, both psychological and physiological, which is the reason why patients usually have elevated cortisol levels[178]. Cortisol is a steroid hormone produced in the adrenal glands during stress.

Excessive cortisol production from the adrenals suppresses the immune system and is therefore harmful to someone who already has a suppressed immune system. Raised cortisol levels specifically raises the TH-2 arm of the immune response, which correlates with auto-immune dysfunction.

Cortisol levels can be reduced with supplementation of DHEA (two tablets first thing in the morning with the same dose repeated 1 h before dinner, on an empty stomach); Melatonin (3 mg sublingually, before bedtime); and Vitamin C (3 daily, in divided doses).

WHAT ARE THE OPTIONS FOR THE FUTURE?

Currently there are three major classes of drugs available for the treatment of AIDS: the nucleoside analog reverse transcriptase inhibitors; the non-nucleoside reverse transcriptase inhibitors; and the HIV protease inhibitors.

When these drugs appeared in the early 1990s, they were shown to reduce death rates in people with AIDS in the short term[198], as they reduced the rate of viral replication and retarded the development of the disease. However, HIV is rapidly developing resistance to these drugs and, as with all drugs, these have side effects, which may be serious in the long term.

DRUG RESISTANCE

One result has been the development of drug-resistant strains of the HI virus that are now rapidly spreading among sexually active individuals in many countries. A study in New York has analysed 80 HIV-positive subjects who had been infected, on average, for less than two months. This meant that they should still have had the original HI virus strain. It was found, however, that 13 of these patients (16%) had genotypes (gene compositions) that were drug resistant. Viruses that were resistant to the reverse transcriptase inhibitors were found in 10 of these patients, while six had viruses that were resistant to protease inhibitors. Multiresistant viruses were found in three of these patients.

This has demonstrated that despite drug treatment, people who were not using condoms were therefore transmitting the resistant viral strains to their sexual partners. Moreover, the viruses that are being passed on are drug resistant. Already there is evidence in the USA of a strain of HIV that is completely resistant to all available anti-AIDS drugs[155]. One alarming characteristic of such resistant viruses is that the patients infected with these viruses rapidly develop full-blown AIDS.

The problem may get far worse as the use of drugs for HIV becomes more widespread and is adopted on a large scale in the developing world.

If AIDS is strictly the result of an infection with a virus only, then the logical approach is to treat and prevent the disease by the elimination of the virus, either by means of a drug or a vaccine. However, these approaches are unlikely to succeed, at least in the foreseeable future, and worse still, there is every likelihood that they will aggravate the problem in the longer term.

VACCINE TRIALS

It is a sobering thought that medical research and practice is largely determined by research funding provided by private pharmaceutical firms who have financial profits in mind. This is illustrated by the history of the development of anti-AIDS vaccines.

Since 1990 funding for the development of new vaccines has increased 600%, and in 2002, $356 million was earmarked for this purpose. Successful experiments in animals have given impetus to this process, with the result that some 25 new vaccines were presented to the AIDS Vaccine Conference in Vancouver in 2001[200]. Currently one is being tested on humans, having progressed from animal studies.

However, some scientists warn against the premature and hasty introduction of new vaccines as they may have irreversible and serious long-term negative consequences.

Dr V Veljkovic, of the Institute of Nuclear Sciences, Belgrade, is one such scientist. He writes that 'despite the urgent need for preventative vaccines, it would be wise to introduce a moratorium on clinical trials until there is a serious re-examination of the current concepts for their development. Premature testing, without complete knowledge of the biological and immunological properties of HIV, could produce irreparable and irreversible long-term consequences.'

What this means is that there is a chance that we may produce vaccine-induced mutations, against which we have no treatment!

The principal obstacle to the development of a successful vaccine (or for that matter a drug) is the fact that HIV has the ability to produce a virtually unlimited number of new strains, of which the more resistant ones to any particular therapy are the ones that will proliferate to infect future hosts[170].

Another problem is the ability of the virus to enter resting T-cells where it may 'hide' for long periods undetected and beyond the reach of drugs or vaccines. Patients inoculated with such a vaccine may appear to have protection against the virus when, in fact, they do not[170].

Dr A Sabin, the developer of the polio vaccine, has doubts about the current prospects of successfully developing an anti-AIDS vaccine. He writes that [203] 'the available data provides no basis for testing any experimental vaccine in human beings or for expecting that any HIV-vaccine could be effective in human beings...

'The vaccines developed for polio and measles are effective because they were directed against viruses that are not attached to cells.' This is in contrast to HIV, which hides inside cells while transferring its genetic code into the DNA genetic material of the host.

However, the difficulties awaiting a vaccine go far beyond the scientific arguments. Such a vaccine will have to be given to hundreds of millions of people, many of whom are HIV-positive. Those given the vaccine may be under the illusion that they are free of the disease while in fact they will still be able to pass on the virus to subsequent generations of sexual partners who are not yet vaccinated. Neither drugs nor vaccines can ever eliminate the virus.

Clearly, the solution does not lie in expensive new drugs and vaccines.

NUTRITIONAL STRATEGIES

Adding selenium to the diet

While there are no examples of the successful use of drugs or vaccines to curb the pandemic, there is at least one good example of how the increased intake of selenium has led to dramatic resistance to HIV, and another where administration of selenium has led to a significant reduction in the level of infection of a virus very similar to HI virus. These are the low incidence of AIDS in Senegal and the successful campaign in China against Keshan disease by the application of selenium supplements.

The pandemic can be largely controlled in southern Africa by enriching the soil with selenium and by taking supplementation.

Soil enrichment with selenium

The methods used by the Chinese include spraying selenium-enriched fertilisers onto soils and crops, adding selenium to the feed of livestock and by adding selenium to salt.

As the level of selenium intake in the local diets increased, the incidence and mortality due to Keshan disease declined[183]. Of course these studies on Keshan disease do not prove that the same thing will happen with HIV and AIDS, which at the time did not occur in China in the areas concerned.

However, both the Coxsackie virus (responsible for Keshan disease) and HIV encode the selenium-containing enzyme glutathione peroxide, making the likelihood that HIV will react in a similar manner extremely strong.

Supplementation

Cost-effective supplements in the form of tablets or capsules are an obvious alternative approach which will have the advantage of yielding practically immediate results.

In contrast to drugs and vaccines, selenium supplementation has the advantage that it will bring long-term relief to those already infected with the virus.

A NOTE ON SELENIUM TOXICITY

Textbooks and publications teach that selenium is toxic when taken in excessive amounts. This is undoubtedly true, but the whole matter has been overemphasised.

Firstly, the symptoms of chronic selenium toxicity are distinctive and easily recognisable, and include brittle hair and fingernails, garlic odour of the breath and a metallic taste in the mouth.

These symptoms are not serious and are easily reversible when selenium intake is reduced or temporarily discontinued.

Not much information is available in the literature on selenium toxicity, presumably because under ordinary circumstances of supplementation and dietary intake, toxicity very rarely occurs.

There are reports of people whose selenium intake is much higher than the usually accepted safe limits (below 800 mcg per day) without any evidence of toxicity symptoms.

One such study conducted in Greenland found a daily intake of selenium in excess of 1 000 mcg daily by the local inhabitants for extended periods of time without any symptoms of toxicity. Presumably the high intake came from local fish sources.

An extreme case has been described in China[176] where local villagers in a region with a very high soil selenium content were tested. The outbreak of toxicity was triggered by the decision to use lime and plant ash fertilisers where the solubility of the soil selenium deposits was greatly increased. As a result the villagers consumed 38 mg (3 800 mcg) of selenium daily, often over lengthy periods of time. Exceptionally high selenium levels were measured in blood, hair, urine and food samples. While the elevated selenium levels killed livestock in the area, the consequences in humans were not so drastic. Exposed patients lost hair and nails, suffered skin lesions, central nervous system and gastro-intestinal disturbances. No deaths occurred and there were no indications of reduced life spans in the elderly.

A FINAL WORD

In evaluating the options available to us in dealing with HIV and AIDS, we will do well to consider our experience in dealing with other major killer diseases such as cancer and heart disease.

There are those in the medical profession who behave as though there is no means of addressing these diseases other than through drug intervention. Since 1971, when the then USA's president Nixon declared war on cancer, they have been searching for the magic bullet that will kill all cancer cells. In 1971, Nixon predicted that by 1976 a solution to the cancer problem, in the form of a super drug, would have been found. Thirty years later, the cancer problem is worse than ever. The truth is that the standard drug-based medical approach to global health problems of this nature has failed.

And now we have the AIDS pandemic. The scientific establishment, guided by medical specialists, has spent more than $40 billion during the last 20 years on research. This research has been based on the assumption that HIV is the sole cause of AIDS, and that if a super drug can be found that will kill the virus, the problem will be solved.

In spite of this massive effort, we are today no nearer to a solution of the problem than we were 20 years ago.

The good news is that during the last number of years, a growing minority of scientists and medical doctors are beginning to see that our past failures are at least partly due to the bias against nutritional intervention in these diseases. But such fundamental changes as are required in the present situation do not come easily, and they do not come without the investment of great effort and persistence.

CHAPTER SIX

CHEMOTHERAPY – OR NOT

Chemotherapy uses chemical compounds (drugs) designed to harm cancer cells more than they harm the host's normal cells. This ideal is difficult to achieve, and invariably some of the normal cells are also damaged. These toxic compounds therefore have to be used judiciously in order to achieve the desired goal.

The idea of finding the 'Achilles Heel' of cancer cells and exploiting it for therapeutic purposes is not an unreasonable one, though, because there are indeed metabolic and other differences between normal and cancer cells. One example is the fact that cancer cells derive their energy mainly from anaerobic metabolism (energy production from carbohydrate and fat fuels without the consumption of oxygen), while normal cells derive energy mainly through the use of oxygen.

Thus if we were able to create an aerobic (oxygen-rich) environment within the body, cancer cells would be at a relative disadvantage compared to the normal cells.

Unfortunately, however, the focus within the development of cancer drugs has not been on exploiting the differences between cancer and normal cells, but rather on the production of toxic substances. Many of these substances are by-products of chemical warfare compounds (such as mustard gas) developed during the two world wars, and originally designed with the opposite objective in mind – to kill normal cells as effectively as possible.

Such highly poisonous drugs (chemotherapeutic agents) are now routinely used in the treatment of at least 70% of all cancer patients, either alone or in combination with treatments such as radiotherapy and surgery[207]. In many cases the results of such treatments have been disastrous.

Dr Abel, a scientist from the Heidelberg Tumor Centre in Germany, has published a comprehensive survey on the world literature on chemotherapy-treated cancer patients[207]. This study shows that among people with epithelial cell cancers (lung, colon, breast and prostate cancers), only 3% survive after chemotherapy.

Nevertheless, chemotherapy does extend survival in many cases of ovarian cancer and in small-cell lung cancer – there seems to be a survival benefit of several months, according to Dr Moss in his book *Questioning Chemotherapy*[211]. In addition, chemotherapy has been successfully used in the treatment of acute anaplastic tumours (childhood leukemia, testicular cancer, Hodgkin's disease) and some other rare cancers, but unfortunately these are perhaps only 5% of all cancers.

In the case of the other 95% of cancers, it is doubtful whether this treatment offers any real advantage. The short-term success rate is about one in five, and even this 'success rate' is short-lived in the case of most tumours. It is true, though, that without chemotherapy this would have been a five in five death rate!

Often the side effects associated with chemotherapy severely affect the quality of a patient's life, raising the question of whether the gains are worthwhile. Some of these are heart muscle and gastro-intestinal damage, nausea, anemia, hair loss and, most importantly, a not readily detectable severe suppression of the immune system.

Dr Bjorksten, an American oncologist, has shown that the immune system may be destroyed irreversibly. This increases the risk that the patient may therefore die of new metastatic cancerous growths, or even of opportunistic infections[208].

Although the functional status of the immune system may be monitored during treatment and dosage levels adjusted accordingly, the currently available detection methods do not monitor all aspects of the immune system and efficacy remains questionable. Dosage limitations arising from such immune monitoring automatically reduce the maximum dosages of chemotherapeutic drugs to a level that may render the treatment ineffective.

The most important weapon anyone has against the proliferation and spreading of cancer is a vigorously active immune system. The natural killer cells of the immune system destroy spreading cancer cells at an early stage, before they have gained a foothold to start new growths elsewhere in the body. Moreover, there is nowhere in the body where cancer cells can 'hide' in order to escape destruction by the immune system; the immune system will find them wherever they are, while chemotherapy drugs do not have access to all of their hiding places, such as the spleen. Furthermore, many of these side effects may be more serious than the disease being treated. In one example, an article in the *New England Journal of Medicine*[239] notes that the risk of developing leukemia as a result of chemotherapy treatment of ovarian cancer outweighs the possible benefit of the treatment. Ironically, leukemia is one of the cancers that can be treated with a degree of success by means of chemotherapy.

Over a period of 90 years, cancer deaths, as a percentage of total mortality, increased from 3,4% in the year 1900 to 25% in 1990; at present it is approaching 30%. Currently, cancer is second only to cardiovascular disease as a cause of death in the developed world; cardiovascular disease is responsible for around 30% of deaths, but will soon take second place to cancer.

In the developed world, the cancer death rate has increased by 50% since 1950; that of prostate cancer by 100%; and that of breast and colon cancer by 60%.

While today approximately one in four people will die of cancer in the developed world, every second person will die of cancer in the year 2017, a mere 13 years from now[209]. This despite $40 billion spent on research and $1 trillion on therapy.

Clearly we are losing the war on cancer, and present treatments, especially chemotherapy, have failed.

WHERE HAVE WE GONE WRONG?

PREVENTION
The medical profession has, on the whole, disregarded the fact that cancer is a disease that can be fairly easily prevented. In 1984, cancer experts from Harvard University presented evidence in the *New England Journal of Medicine* that 90% of all cancers are environmentally induced, and therefore preventable[210]. This is confirmed by the fact that the incidence of cancer in primitive societies and many developing countries is extremely low.

However as soon as people adopt a Western lifestyle and diet, cancer incidence rises. This demonstrates that prevention by means of lifestyle and dietary changes are far superior to any wonder drug (which is, in any case, unlikely to materialise).

The problem, however, is that it is extremely difficult to convince people to change their harmful habits. Most of us are comfort-orientated, so changing our way of life calls for some effort, and we'll only make these changes if we have a deep conviction that such changes are really necessary. This is hampered to a large extent by the budgets and persuasive tactics of groups who'd rather we didn't change, such as those who sell cigarettes and refined foods.

MISLEADING REPORTS

The popular press is always ready to sensationalise reports of every new drug that appears, whether or not such a drug has been properly evaluated.

As each miracle drug appears on the scene, the previous one is forgotten...

Unfortunately, certain sections of the medical profession and specifically the cancer research establishment are not without blame.

These misleading reports often create confusion among the general public and furthermore perpetuate the idea that the solution lies in the imminent development of a new drug. This creates an atmosphere of expectation in the minds of many cancer patients, whilst at the same time discrediting those few cases where chemotherapy has merit.

EVALUATION OF CANCER DRUGS

Some chemotherapeutic agents do have an effect on the course of cancer development, reported as 'tumour shrinkage', 'responses', 'reduced cancer activity', 'progression-free' or even 'disease-free' by researchers.

The question is whether any of these have any real practical value for the patient who is interested in long-term survival, with a similar quality of life to that before he or she was diagnosed with cancer.

The survival of those few patients who do live longer than the magical five-year point noted in clinical trials is bought at the expense not only of their own quality of life but of all the other patients who are similarly treated and who do not benefit. It is important to distinguish between survival (for example, living for five years after treatment), and cure.

These considerations have prompted Dr Abel to remark that arguing for the benefit of chemotherapy based on the few successes is like arguing in favour of gambling based on the profits of one or a few winners[211].

Another cancer researcher, oncologist Dr A Braverman of New York, has expressed similar sentiments. He points out that 'many oncologists recommend chemotherapy for virtually any tumour with a hopefulness undiscouraged by almost invariable failure'. He calls on doctors to 'scale back the whole chemotherapeutic enterprise'[212].

WHEN YOUR DOCTOR GETS CANCER...

There have been a number of studies that have investigated this intriguing question. The most important and most rigorous of these was carried out at McGill University in 1993 and involved the treatment of patients with non-small-cell lung cancer, a type of cancer for which[213] chemotherapy is frequently prescribed.

The Canadian Cancer Centre at the University sent out a questionnaire to 118 practicing oncologists who treat non-small-cell lung cancer. These doctors recruited patients for treatment in the normal course of work, then participated in clinical trials based on this treatment. For these clinical trials, the doctors were asked to imagine that they themselves had non-small-cell lung cancer and were then asked to indicate which of different on-going clinical trials (reflecting different treatment modalities) they would join. The answers were illuminating.

A large percentage (81%) of those specialists who responded and who every day treated other people with this type of cancer would not consent to participate as patients in any of the trials in which chemotherapy treatment was used. Seventy three percent specifically refused to be treated with cisplatin, a chemotherapeutic agent noted for its high degree of toxicity. The main reasons given for these answers were the ineffectiveness of chemotherapy and its associated toxicity.

These answers reflect a shocking degree of hypocrisy on the part of these specialists, although it is true that there are no studies that indicate what oncologists actually do do when they have cancer – their behaviour could differ from their survey answers. The survey also revealed that the more patients a particular doctor treated per year, the less inclined he was to participate as a patient in a trial.

Supporting evidence comes from other specialists in the field. Dr H Hansen from the Finsen Institute in Copenhagen, Denmark, also a trialist in chemotherapeutic trials, wrote in an editorial in the *Journal of Clinical Oncology* in 1987: 'Based on the literature, it is difficult not to concur with our colleagues in not taking treatments. One can question the justification of continuing therapeutic trials along these lines in non-small-cell lung cancer'[214].

Dr Abel came to a similar conclusion as a result of his own international survey. Based on the replies to a letter sent to oncologists in numerous countries, he found that 'the personal views of many oncologists seem to be in striking contrast to communications intended for the public'[215].

WHY THE BIAS TOWARD CHEMOTHERAPY?

Medical policy is decided at meetings of specific disease committees or at so-called 'consensus conferences', called by the medical bodies representing the medical profession. Frequently, such meetings are steered in a specific direction by one or more 'opinion-formers', who are at times motivated more by concerns of personal prestige and financial reward than scientific merit. Standard treatment procedures evolve from such meetings, and are referred to as 'standard treatment protocols', which all doctors are expected to follow. Doctors who fail to do so may risk prosecution for malpractice.

Such meetings are frequently aimed at improving (by fine adjustments) the use of existing chemotherapeutic agents rather than considering viable alternatives to the use of chemotherapeutic agents. This is the level at which financial interests get a foot in the door, and so often succeed in steering medical thinking.

THE MAJOR BIASES

The most respected evaluation method, the placebo-controlled double-blind clinical trial, offers the least opportunity for error and bias, but certain distortions may still – willingly or accidentally – be introduced. In this type of trial, patients are randomly allocated into two equal groups. One group is given the active medication (for example, the chemotherapy drug) while the other group is given an inactive drug that is identical in appearance. The trial is known as 'double-blinded' when neither the researcher nor the trialists know which is the active preparation.

One way in which the results of such a trial could be distorted takes place during the statistical evaluation of the trial, where findings are sometimes reported only on the 'evaluable' patients rather than on all the patients who entered the trial or study.

For example, those who fare the worst may be removed from the trial (for ethical or other reasons) because they could not tolerate the full treatment for a sufficient length of time. This introduces a distortion that makes the treatment seem more effective.

Another bias creeps in when survival times are given only for the responders, whilst nothing is said about the non-responders.

Then there are those cases where the authors have a financial stake in the outcome of the trial. There is no question that some oncologists are influenced by their financial involvement in the drugs they evaluate or recommend, and it is not impossible to find out which trialists are taking placebos and which the active drugs. This problem may be much larger that most of us would have expected. Dr D Kessler, Commissioner of the US Food and Drug Administration in 1997, is one of the few who expresses his reservations in this regard. 'Everything is tainted,' he says. 'Almost every doctor in academia has something going on the side, and I don't know what it is and I don't have the authority to find out. I don't know what they are getting legally as far as financial return, stock, money whatever. I certainly don't know what they are getting under the table'[212].

Most ordinary doctors and oncologists are probably not guilty of such misconduct, but since they have to abide by policies and since they are not in a position to scientifically evaluate specific treatments on their own, they usually follow what is prescribed by the cancer establishment. This is the mechanism by which the interests of the big companies reach the general public, and therefore the lucrative market of chemotherapeutic drugs.

It is unfortunately not possible to conduct meaningful clinical studies with drugs (conducted and paid for mostly by the pharmaceutical companies) without involving and paying medical specialists (in this case oncologists). In some cases, the situation is legitimate. The problem arises when the drug to be tested does not perform as well as was hoped for, and certain 'adjustments' to the data are required. This is when the statistics are limited to 'evaluable patients' or otherwise manoeuvered to improve the picture.

At worst, such a conflict of interest may spiral into outright fraud, as was pointed out by Dr R Smith, the editor of the *British Medical Journal*. In 1998 he noted that 'research misconduct is like child abuse. Once you recognise it, you start to see there's a lot of it about...'.

Fraud includes fabricating or inventing data – at least one such case is on record, in a much-celebrated clinical trial of high-dose chemotherapy with bone marrow transplantation in breast cancer[211].

Other less clear cases involve the 'drenching' of data when a clinical trial turns out negative. In such cases, the researchers search the data for possible subgroups in the study population that appear to have benefited from the treatment. For example, in the treatment of breast cancer patients with chemotherapy, a subgroup may be identified (eg consumers of alcohol between the ages of 50 and 60) that have benefited from the treatment. There is nothing wrong with searching for such subgroups, provided they are significant and that they do materially benefit patients. However, this is often not the case. Some researchers then write up the trial as though it was originally designed to study only this subgroup, creating an altogether false impression of the value of the drug.

Another factor that makes a trial look better than it actually is, relates to improvements in diagnostic technology that make the diagnosis of cancer possible at an earlier stage than it was 20–30 years ago. The 'statistical life' of patients in a clinical trial is extended, making it look as though the patients have lived longer when in fact they did not. They were simply diagnosed earlier.

Such a fallacy is responsible for current claims that we can now handle breast cancer better than we could 20 years ago. In spite of the fact that it is now widely recognised, some researchers still commit this error, and it has been responsible for some false claims about the effectiveness of chemotherapy.

Publication bias is another error that contributes to false conclusions – trials that claim positive results are more readily published than those that do not. After a while, the published studies on the usefulness of a particular chemotherapy drug which reflect a positive result greatly outnumber those that have produced negative results, creating an illusion of the drug's superiority.

Often unintentional, these errors can also be the result of peer pressure (trialists want to produce 'results' in a highly competitive field) and financial gain. Another factor is personal prestige and the feeling of 'being one of the leaders'. In order to achieve this, study directors must produce positive results in clinical trials, and money for trials is always necessary. There is therefore enormous pressure to please their research sponsors.

These factors that distort the results of otherwise good clinical trials are far more common than suspected, because most of us do not have the background and training necessary to recognise them when they occur.

Collectively they are the reason why patients and even doctors believe that a particular treatment has more merit than it actually has.

FINANCIAL INCENTIVES

Most of us assume that our doctors will select for us the very best treatment available, and that the drugs they prescribe are the best ones for the purpose. In many instances this trust is indeed justified, but in other instances unfortunately it is not.

The international market for chemotherapy drugs is huge, worth billions of dollars per year. Estimates of the number of people receiving chemotherapy treatment each year varies from 300 000 to one million in the USA alone[211], and these only refer to recorded hospital admissions! Many patients are treated with chemotherapy outside formal institutions.

What about the cost per patient?

Chemotherapy drugs are expensive, and in the case of some of the newer drugs, these costs can be prohibitive. Estimates of drugs costs alone (excluding physician's fees, hospitalisation, etc) for a course of standard drug treatment for breast cancer vary from $5 000 to $25 000 in the USA.

At least one case was highlighted in the American press in 1991: a woman who was treated for chronic granulocytic leukemia for two years with chemotherapy, full body radiation and bone marrow transplantation. When she died her unpaid medical bills amounted to $600 000.

Today the annual expenditure on cancer drugs is well in excess of $14 billion.

But what are the benefits? In most cases patients live a few months longer, during which time they often have to endure severe side effects.

Many leading cancer specialists promote chemotherapy for virtually every cancer type, without considering the real benefits and whether, by using much cheaper and simpler treatments such as high-dose vitamin C, the patients would not be better served.

WORLDWIDE CANCER CHEMOTHERAPY MARKET REVENUE FORECASTS
*WITH REFERENCE TO THE PREVIOUS YEAR

YEAR	REVENUE ($ MILLION)	REVENUE GROWTH RATE(%)(*)
1990	3 531	13,7
1995	8 591	14,3
1999	13 790	12,1

The compound annual growth rate over the period 1992–1999 was 13,1%.
SOURCE: market intelligence company Frost & Sullivan

WHAT'S THE PAYOFF?

Swedish scientist Prof B Jonssen has devoted his attention to looking at the benefits of this financial outlay, but reports that little direct evidence is available by way of clinical trial analysis. He does present some information from the 'notional patient benefit year' (NPBY), an index designed by economists as a measure to express health care costs.

NPBY index is the cost that society (patients and insurers) pays for each year of cancer-free survival achieved by any specific treatment. Thus the least effective treatments will have the highest NPBY costs. The following table has been adapted from information by Dr Jonssen[216]:

TREATMENT	NPBY COSTS ($)
Chemotherapy for advanced, previously treated non-small-cell lung cancer with vindesine, etoposide and cisplatin	174 720
Chemotherapy for metastatic non-small-cell lung cancer (cyclophosphamide, doxorubicin, etoposide)	28 080
Tamoxifen for advanced breast cancer	593
Chemotherapy for metastatic teratoma	172

RELATIVE VALUES OF CANCER TREATMENTS

Chemotherapy, when it is truly effective (such as in the treatment of testicular cancer), is a relatively cheap option. In most cases it is a costly treatment due to the short survival time and high cost of the drugs.

THE ROLE OF DRUG COMPANIES

Considering the size of the market, and its expansion rate, it is not surprising that the pharmaceutical giants have a keen interest in chemotherapy. These companies invest huge sums of money towards the development of new drugs.

Bristol-Myers Squibb, for example, spends $1 billion per year on research and employs 4 000 scientists and supporting personnel[217]. Other large pharmaceutical manufacturers have similar large budgets devoted to research.

Collectively, these companies provide a considerable portion of the total cancer research effort. Although their involvement does have its downside, this research is not without great benefit to humanity. Where else would such large sums of money for research be found? Society's needs for new treatments are indeed reflected in the budgets of these companies, and they, in turn, respond because they expect and reap huge financial rewards.

These companies also creatively influence cancer research in other spheres. They support research projects at universities and they make available a variety of grants that are invaluable in sustaining growth and development in cancer research.

However, it is essential to grasp that these companies consider the cancer problem as a business venture, which they tend to develop and steer towards their own financial ends ('the cancer industry'). Thus the greatest impetus is not necessarily given to avenues of research that are the most rewarding to the patients but rather to what they consider will bring the greatest rewards.

Because of their powerful research effort, drug companies have managed to infiltrate research institutions such as the Sloan-Kettering Institute in New York. Such influence is not necessarily unethical, but by its very presence, it has had a decisive influence on medical thinking, which has not always been in the best interests of the patient. During the last 15 years both the chair and vice-chair of the board of Sloan-Kettering were directors of Bristol-Myers.

The result has been that research institutions in the USA have maintained a strong prochemotherapy stance, which has unavoidably filtered through to doctors and practising oncologists.

It is not unreasonable to ask to whose benefit is the war on cancer being fought?

To some extent the patient may benefit, but the major benefits (financial) go to the drug companies and the doctors who administer them.

Even the editor of the *Journal of the American Medical Association* remarked at a meeting of the government-sponsored National Institutes of Health in 1995 that 'efforts by those with vested interests to influence decision-makers to use their power are ever more creative; efforts by manufacturers to influence publications that position their products in as favourable a light as possible are pervasive and frequently well-disguised... It is a marvelous opportunity for rampant deceit. So much money is there to be made that ethical principles can be overrun, sometimes in a stampede to get at physicians and prescribers'[218].

There is no question that many well-meaning doctors are misled by scientific papers that express unwarranted and misplaced optimism about chemotherapy. Many doctors fail to inform patients about the lack of evidence of long-term benefit to the patient.

DOES CHEMOTHERAPY EVER WORK?

It is astonishing that critical questions are seldom asked and seldom addressed. The least one could expect scientifically minded doctors to ask are the basic questions: 'Is it any better than placebo (good, supportive care)? Does it have a positive effect on patient survival (and, if so, how much)?'

Frequently patients are told that the 'newer generation' of chemotherapeutic agents are more effective and less toxic than the older ones. I have not been able to find any firm evidence in support of such claims. Often these claims are based on evidence that is unrelated to real patient benefit in terms of survival: for example, tumour shrinkage is not synonymous with survival!

BREAST CANCER

Dr Moss has concluded that 'complete remissions [of breast cancer] are rare and in any case do not correlate with increased survival. In fact there is no evidence that survival is actually improved by chemotherapy'[211].

Such a conclusion is in accordance with a large volume of anecdotal evidence[220]. There are few people who do not know of a friend or relative with breast cancer who died after receiving treatment with chemotherapeutic drugs. It is true that patients may live longer after treatment, but complete long-term cures are seldom achieved.

PROSTATE CANCER

This is the most common type of cancer in men in the developing world. It also has certain features not seen in other types of cancer.

Most men with prostate cancer will die from other diseases without knowing that they ever had prostate cancer[220], and 40% of all men over 50 have latent prostate cancer. Up to 67% of elderly men who died of other causes have been found to have prostate cancer.

Prostate cancers are often slow-growing. In advanced cancer of the prostate, hormone blockage therapy is used. The problem is that after several years, these cancers may become resistant to hormone modulating therapy. The use of hormone modulating agents on an intermittent basis prolongs the time before this happens[45]. The precise role and efficacy of chemotherapy in the treatment of prostate cancer remains undefined[221].

However, through improved diagnostic procedures doctors can now find small pockets of cancer cells that would not have been detected formerly, but fewer than 10% of such tumours ever develop to the point of clinical significance. Thus, the 'increased survival rates' are simply due to the fact that greater numbers of insignificant 'cancers' are now detected and 'cured'. Such treatments will not save lives but will increase the number of patients who 'survive'.

LUNG CANCERS

Small-cell lung cancer is of particular interest because it is one of the very few cancers of epithelial tissue in which there is evidence of increased survival after chemotherapy. This increased survival is limited to weeks and at the most a few months, though.

A typical example is that of a placebo-controlled trial in which chemotherapy treatment was compared with placebo. The placebo group had an average survival of 42 days while the treated group lived for 110 days. The trialists would therefore have been justified in claiming that chemotherapy prolonged survival by nearly 300%. Sometimes results such as these are reported in the popular press with much fanfare. What they omit to say is that the patients only survived for a little more than three months, and for that small benefit they had to pay a heavy price, not only financially, but also in terms of severe side effects.

The side effects of chemotherapy drugs, especially when used in high concentrations and in combinations with other drugs, are severe. In some studies, up to two thirds of patients had life-threatening toxicity and some have died toxic deaths from the treatment itself. There is also no evidence that combination therapy involving chemotherapy is any better than single agent treatment.

The average survival time in a trial in 1976 with a large group of people with terminal small-cell lung cancer (for which all forms of treatment, including chemotherapy, had been abandoned), treated with high-dose vitamin C, was 300 days longer than the untreated controls[45].

With non-small-cell lung cancer, there may be weak indications of a life-prolonging effect of the chemotherapy drug, cisplatin. These effects are quite small, though, and are paid for heavily in terms of toxicity.

Six double-blind placebo-controlled studies have taken place in which chemotherapy was compared with the best supportive care as alternative. The use of chemotherapy resulted in a survival gain of 1,1 months, which increased to 2,3 months when cisplatin was added, but this additional advantage was purchased at great cost in terms of severe side effects[223], such as liver and kidney damage.

OTHER TYPES OF CANCER

In some of the relatively rare kinds of cancer, such as childhood leukemia and testicular cancer, chemotherapy has been shown to be of value, and in some cases may even effect a cure. Unfortunately these are kinds of cancer mostly seen in children and young adults. Moreover, the list of cancers that are responsive to chemotherapy has virtually remained unchanged over the past 30 years.

The list of cancers for which chemotherapy treatment has definite benefits include acute lymphocytic leukemia, Hodgkin's disease and some other lymphomas (eg Burkitts lymphoma) and testicular cancer.

As for the many other solid cancers in adults, there is no compelling direct or even indirect evidence of benefit nor any proof that such treatment improves the quality of life.

REDUCING THE SIDE EFFECTS AND IMPROVING EFFICACY OF CHEMO

Vitamins, and especially the antioxidants, have been found to interact favourably with chemotherapeutic agents.

A considerable body of clinical evidence shows that such vitamin supplements not only enhance the efficacy of chemotherapeutic agents but, at the same time, also reduce toxic side effects[45].

High-dose vitamin C prolongs the life of terminal cancer patients more efficiently than most chemotherapeutic agents (see page 118).

Linus Pauling (scientist and winner of Nobel prizes for biochemistry and peace) has noted that 'vitamin C ...controls to a considerable extent the disagreeable side effects of the cytotoxic chemotherapeutic agents, such as nausea and loss of hair, and that benefit seems to add its value to that of the chemotherapeutic agents. We now recommend a high intake of vitamin C, in some cases up to the bowel tolerance limit, beginning as early as possible'[224].

Furthermore, when vitamin C is used in conjunction with chemotherapy drugs, it has been shown to reduce the toxicity of the drugs significantly in several studies. This means that higher doses of the chemotherapy could be used, making them more effective – all chemotherapy drugs would work better if we could use higher concentrations, but toxicity prohibits this. People with terminal cancer have extremely low vitamin C blood levels, to the extent that they may develop scurvy[45]. This seriously compromises the patient's immunocompetence at a time when it is of really great importance to survival[226].

CHEMOTHERAPY-INDUCED VITAMIN DEFICIENCIES

Patients on chemotherapy drugs may develop serious vitamin deficiencies, which include vitamins B1, B2, B3, C, folic acid and vitamin K. Logically such deficiencies could be very harmful (including detrimental effects on the immune system which is of utmost importance to the cancer patient)[225].

Vitamin C, for example, increases the cancer cell killing capacity of chemotherapy[226], and in animal experiments vitamin E reduced the toxicity of certain chemotherapeutic agents. Since bone marrow transplantation depletes vitamin E in patients, it has been suggested that this could partly explain the toxicity associated with the procedure.

There is no question that antioxidants are important in both bone marrow transplant patients as well as those being treated with chemotherapeutic drugs. For this reason German doctors have suggested high-dose supplementation of essential antioxidants such as vitamins E and C in patients undergoing bone marrow transplantation.

In spite of this and other supporting evidence[45], many doctors still advise their patients not to take vitamin supplements while on chemotherapy treatment. The argument is that by reducing the toxicity of these drugs, the vitamins also reduce the efficacy of the treatment.

There are now dozens of studies that prove exactly the opposite[45]. These studies show that instead of decreasing the efficacy of chemotherapy, they actually increase it. Vitamin and mineral supplements enhance the killing capacity of these drugs.

It is considered that some vitamins and minerals, used in conjunction with chemotherapy, will protect normal tissues and potentiate the destruction of cancer cells. For example, studies done at the National Cancer Institute in America have shown that antioxidants do protect the hearts of patients receiving doxorubicin (adriamycin), a well-known cardiotoxic drug, without interfering with its ability to kill cancer cells[227].

THE POTENTIAL OF VITAMIN C

In the 1970s Dr E Cameron (oncologist) and Dr L Pauling conducted trials with high dose vitamin C on terminally ill cancer patients in the Vale of Leven hospital in Scotland, where up to 4 000 such patients are under treatment and care.

Large numbers of cancer patients (various types of cancer) participated in the trials in which survival times in vitamin C treated cancer patients were compared with those in an appropriately selected control group. Both overall cancer mortality as well as cancer deaths due to specific types of cancer were documented, which yielded a wealth of information. Details are available in the excellent book by Cameron and Pauling[229].

One of the most important conclusions they reached is the strong evidence that treatment of terminally ill cancer patients (in whom conventional treatments including chemotherapy had failed) with 10 g of vitamin C daily increased survival time by approximately 300 days on average. Some patients lived for much longer, and 5% appear to have been cured completely – they were still alive five years later.

All types of cancer responded, but bladder, breast, kidney and colon cancers responded best.

There is little doubt that a high intake of vitamin C is beneficial to most people with advanced cancer, with greatly improved quality of life being a conspicuous feature.

All experiments were conducted on people with terminal cancer in whom conventional treatment methods, including chemotherapy, were no longer effective. It is quite possible that treatment with high-dose vitamin C at an earlier stage, before chemotherapy, could have been even more successful. In that sense, the trials did not constitute (nor were they intended) to be a direct comparison of the relative value of chemotherapy and high-dose vitamin C in the management of cancer patients.

THE WAY FORWARD

An unbiased evaluation of chemotherapeutic drugs is hampered by the involvement of the big pharmaceutical companies which, while rendering valuable support to cancer research on the one hand, unavoidably also influence the course of research and ultimately medical thinking as a result of their huge financial involvement in cancer research.

However, there is firm evidence to support the use of chemotherapy in the treatment of certain cancers, especially in young people (eg acute lymphocytic leukemia, Hodgkin's disease, testicular cancer and a handful of other rare cancers). Unfortunately these cancers constitute only about 5% of all cancers.

Evidence for the life-prolonging effect in the other more common cancers is weak and reflects a gain of life expectancy of weeks to months at best. This slight advantage comes at a high price in terms of financial costs and severe toxicity.

In the case of the majority of other cancers, such proof is simply non-existent.

Authorities appear to be unaware of (or otherwise reluctant to react to) the considerable advantages of high-dose vitamin C in terminally ill cancers, which are much more impressive than those of the chemotherapeutic drugs.

Resorting to chemotherapy without establishing the likelihood of success not only virtually ensures failure but has the additional disadvantage that it reduces the likelihood of benefiting from other less harmful and more promising new treatments, based on nutritional and other treatments that strengthen the immune system[45].

By damaging the bone marrow and the immune system, chemotherapy may seriously reduce the patient's own defence mechanisms which could have facilitated recovery.

In spite of assurances given by oncologists to the contrary, word has spread among the population that chemotherapy is a death sentence, which in many cases, it is.

These are some factors that the patient who contemplates chemotherapy should consider, preferably in consultation with his or her oncologist.

Demand solid, scientific proof of the efficacy of the proposed treatment and establish whether there is at least a reasonable chance of success. Do not be afraid to question your doctor and specifically demand to see the evidence on which the proposed treatment is based. If necessary, enlist the help of a professional friend to interpret results.

Be on your guard against evasive tactics. The most common one is that the proposed treatment is so new that information is not yet available. If it has not yet been evaluated properly, don't take chances with your life. You are not a guinea pig.

Remember there is a 'party line' within the medical profession, which many doctors feel compelled to uphold.

Do not be misled by the type of evidence of efficacy that may be unrelated to patient survival. The only acceptable evidence is positive proof of life extension based on peer-reviewed controlled clinical trials published in prestigious medical journals.

Be sufficiently informed to discuss these matters openly and intelligently with your oncologist. This is not as difficult as it may sound – you don't have to become an oncologist in order to discuss the vitally important points with your oncologists.

Read Dr Moss's publication, *Chemotherapy Questioned*[211]. If your oncologist still belongs to the 'old school' who refuses to discuss the subject on these lines 'because he is the doctor and he should know', then you will be doing yourself a favour by finding another, more enlightened oncologist.

Consider the use of non-toxic, natural treatments that are based on acceptable clinical proof. Such treatments do exist and, in many cases, they are much more effective than chemotherapy[45]. Remember also that orthodox doctors are usually poorly informed on these alternative treatments[228]. For example, don't forget about the importance of high-dose vitamin C.

CHAPTER SEVEN

LIFE - GIVING BACTERIA

Bacteria are not all bad! We cannot live without the 'friendly bacteria' in the human gut, but the 'unfriendly bacteria' that live there either do nothing to promote health or actively cause disease.

Beneficial bacteria are collectively referred to as probiotics. They are life-giving, as opposed to the antibiotics, and health is largely dependent on the balance between these two groups of micro-organisms.

Most people, even health professionals, do not realise the extent to which these micro-organisms are involved in disease, nor the extent to which, in the average person, this balance is less than ideal. The result can be much inconvenience and suffering, and the body becomes prone to many disease states such as constipation, diarrhoea, immune system disorders and even cancers. Yet, too often, neither patient nor doctor is able to pinpoint the cause.

The most important health-promoting properties of probiotic bacteria are the way in which they suppress disease-causing intestinal micro-organisms (bacteria, yeasts) and normalise digestion and gut functions.

They do this, for example, by adhering to the mucous membrane in the gut and by increasing the acidity of the gut to suit their own requirements, while at the same time suppressing the growth of other organisms.

More than a kilogram of mixed organisms in the human gut perform many critical functions, including completing the digestion of food through fermentation, protecting against disease-causing pathogenic micro-organisms such as candida, and, most importantly, maintaining a healthy immune system.

Candida is a yeast-like micro-organism that normally occurs in the gut without causing problems, but under certain conditions it may change and become pathogenic. Apart from gastro-intestinal symptoms, systemic effects of this bacteria are also seen in the urinary system (vaginal and bladder infections), the immune system (repeat infections, allergies, chemical sensitivities), the nervous system (depression, irritability and inability to concentrate) and the hormonal system (PMS-like symptoms).

The most dominant probiotics belong to the lactobacillus and bifidobacteria families. Humans are not born with these gut micro-organisms, but the newborn baby gets a dose of them as it passes through the birth canal during delivery. These bacteria are present in the vaginal secretions, of which babies ingest minute quantities. After this initial dose, these bacteria start to grow in the baby's gut within hours, where they assist with the digestion of mother's milk. It may happen that babies born by C-section have chronic digestive problems because they don't receive this 'dose' at birth, but as they grow they do receive these organisms through food and in contact with other people.

Bifidobacteria infantis is also present in breast milk, and if babies do not get enough of it they may suffer from poor nutrition and allergies. Since these bacteria do not require iron for growth (mother's milk does not contain iron), lactobacillus and bifidobacteria are able to populate the digestive tract at a time when other organisms, which do require iron, are unable to do so, thus preventing the introduction of pathogens at a stage when the baby cannot cope with them.

The lactobacilli and related organisms therefore play a key role in an infant's health, and they continue to do so throughout life.

MAKING THE MOST OF YOUR PROBIOTICS

The efficiency of friendly bacteria may be reduced as a result of stress, disease and poor diet. Alcohol, foreign chemicals, yeasts and a diet high in refined foods and sugars can adversely affect probiotics. They are severely handicapped by certain drugs too, particularly antibiotics and the sulpha drugs. Some antibiotics, even when taken at subtherapeutic levels, can destroy probiotic bacteria. Steroid hormones (cortisone, oral contraceptives and other steroids) severely affect probiotics as well.

Variations in intestinal acidity will also adversely affect the probiotics. Highly alkaline conditions are undesirable, and the most important factors that influence this acidity[149] are stress (presumably as a result of rising cortisone levels) and a refined diet.

The peristaltic activity in the gut also influences the activity of probiotic bacteria. Either way, whether this activity is too rapid (diarrhoea and irritable bowel syndrome) or too slow (constipation), the viability of the intestinal flora is adversely affected. These effects tend to have a multiplying effect: a poor diet reduces probiotic activity, which is further aggravated by the suppressed peristalsis that accompanies a poor diet.

PROBIOTICS AND THE IMMUNE SYSTEM

The mass of probiotic cells in the gut is probably the most important single 'organ' in the body that controls immunocompetence.

The immune system consists of a complicated system of cells and proteins (including antibodies) designed to protect us against external invaders (micro-organisms) as well as aberrant internal cells that may be life endangering (such as cancer cells). The immune cells are formed from primitive stem cells produced in the bone marrow. These cells then mature into different organs and structures to produce a variety of immune cells with specific functions.

Stem cells from the bone marrow differentiate into two types of precursor cells, called lymphocyte precursors and macrophage precursors.

The lymphocyte precursors mature in certain tissues (such as the bone marrow and the spleen) to form what are known as natural killer cells, B-lymphocytes (B-cells) and T-lymphocytes (T-cells). These natural killer cells are scavengers that set out to destroy cancer cells and other large invaders.

The B-lymphocytes produce antibodies that attack invading molecules such as toxins, while the T-lymphocytes also attack the invaders but at the same also time co-ordinate immune function by calling up other immune cells.

The B-cells produce antibodies called immunoglobulins, including immunoglobulin type A (IgA), a secretory antibody produced by the lymphoid tissue in the gut.

The T-cells are also divided into T-helper cells, which enhance the immune response, and T-suppressor cells, which reduce the level of immune response, thus having an overall modulating effect on immune function.

The system functions as an efficient whole, but the lymphocytes (B- and T-) play the leading roles. Lymphocytes are found throughout the tissues of the body, in the blood and lymph, however they accumulate in certain tissues, which are designated as 'lymphoid tissue'. The lymphatic capillaries unite to form lymphatic ducts, which convey the lymph to the lymph nodes where invaders accumulate and are exposed to the immune system cells (which are also concentrated there).

Probiotic bacteria are concentrated in the mucosa-associated lymph tissue (MALT), which is the largest lymphoid tissue mass in the human body[150]. Probiotics and the MALT form an integral part of the body's total immune capacity. The most important consequence of this is the fact that probiotics can elicit and modulate a specific immune response by the enhanced production of IgA antibodies, which protect the body against bacteria, yeasts, fungi and viruses, including the flu virus.

Probiotic bacteria also enhance T-cell function by activating T-helper cells (Th1 and Th2), and promote the maturation development of lymphoid tissue in the gut (GALT).

Finally, they may also stimulate the non-specific immune response based on natural killer cells and macrophages.

PROBIOTICS IN ACTION

DIARRHOEA
Many studies have shown that the administration of probiotics can be dramatically effective in the treatment of this troublesome condition. One study published in 2001 showed that probiotics can be effective against many different kinds of viral diarrhoea, in some case reducing the incidence by 50%[142].

Several studies have shown that lactobacillus preparations can reduce the incidence of diarrhoea in children who are taking antibiotics[143]. In many children the damage done to the microflora (the total microbial population) by the antibiotics is real and serious, and does not manifest as diarrhoea but as severely reduced immunity instead. This results in repeated infections, for which more antibiotics are prescribed; the immune system is further suppressed, and a vicious circle is thus set in motion.

Although many doctors do advise parents to use probiotic supplements in children on antibiotic treatment, the type, timing and doses of such supplements are often wrong, resulting in no beneficial effects being seen. Such supplements should be taken after the period of treatment, otherwise the antibiotics kill or suppress the administered probiotics. Other studies have demonstrated the effectiveness of probiotic treatment in reducing the risk of 'traveller's diarrhoea' and diarrhoea in hospital pediatric wards[143].

CROHN'S DISEASE AND ULCERATIVE COLITIS

In one study on 15 patients with ulcerative colitis, probiotic treatment brought about remission in 12 of them (80%)[144].

Other studies have shown similar positive responses in people with Crohn's disease and irritable bowel syndrome.

ALLERGIES

Diseases that are the result of an allergic response are known as atopic diseases. Typical examples are asthma, eczema and allergic rhinitis. Double-blinded randomised control trials have shown a positive response to probiotic treatment in all of these conditions, where the basic mechanism involved is the important normalising effect probiotics have on the immune system (see below).

One study, published in 2001, used 159 pregnant women with one or more conditions (asthma, eczema, allergic rhinitis) as the sample, and investigated the effect of probiotic treatment on their offspring. The women were subdivided into two equal groups, one of which was treated with probiotics two to four weeks before the expected delivery dates. The babies continued to receive probiotic treatment after birth for six months, when the results of the study were evaluated. These children were all expected to be at high risk for the diseases concerned. By the age of two, the incidence of these diseases in the treated group of babies was only 50% of that in the placebo group[145].

CANCER

Because of the effect probiotics have on the immune system, it is not surprising to find that they have a protective effect against at least some cancers, and that they may be of value in the treatment of cancer.

In animal and laboratory studies, different probiotic strains have been shown to inhibit intestinal, breast, liver and especially colon cancer[146]. In a study published in 2001 in the *Journal of the American Dietetics Association*, evidence was presented that probiotics may lengthen the remission time of bladder cancer.

Probiotics stimulate the B-cells as well as natural killer cells and macrophages against cancer cells. They also stimulate the secretion of the chemical messengers[151] interleukins and cytokines, that destroy cancer cells, and they can remove and 'disarm' procarcinogens in the gut, such as the bile acids.

CHOLESTEROL

Probiotics have been shown to lower raised blood cholesterol levels and help in the control of blood pressure, as they affect the biochemical pathway in the body that leads to the synthesis of cholesterol.

In one double-blinded placebo control trial with lactobacillus sporogenes as a probiotic supplement, total cholesterol was reduced by 32% and LDL cholesterol by 35% in only three months. In the case of lactobacillus acidophilus and bifidobacteria, these claims have not yet been fully substantiated.

WHEN SHOULD YOU TAKE PROBIOTICS?

The answer to this question lies in your diet. A diet rich in refined foods promotes the growth of many pathogens over the healthy bacteria, ultimately resulting in a distorted balance. This may be immediately visible, such as in the case of difficult-to-treat candida infections, but in most cases the harmful effects are present in the patient who feels vaguely 'not well'.

On a diet rich in unrefined, whole foods, however, the gut is able to maintain a healthy balance of microflora all on its own. Such diets provide adequate quantities of natural antibiotics. However, if you have taken a course of antibiotics within the last year, or if you consume alcohol, or if your diet contains a high proportion of refined foods or you take oral contraceptives, consider probiotic supplements of the right kind, whether or not you notice any symptoms.

Faecal consistency is often a good indicator of the condition of the gut flora. In the absence of a healthy bacterial population in the gut, the faeces is often not well formed (diarrhoea tendency) or very hard (constipation). The bacterial population of the healthy colon should consist of at least 80–90% lactobacillus (and related organisms). The rest is mostly gut micro-organisms. In Western populations on a refined diet high in sugar, the bacterial population is often in the reverse ratio. This results in constipation (or sometimes diarrhoea), excessive gas with bloating, intestinal and systemic toxicity, malabsorption of nutrients and overgrowth of harmful yeast (candida).

Sometimes you may be following a healthy diet, yet still have allergies or digestive problems that are a legacy of earlier events. In such instances, or if you have to take antibiotics, drugs or even herbs that work like antibiotics (eg olive leaf extract or golden seal), you may want to consider probiotics. It is also worth considering probiotic treatment if you have recurrent bladder and vaginal infections, to prevent 'traveller's diarrhoea' due to food poisoning or if you have chronic health problems such as asthma, acne or arthritis.

If you have chronic bowel disease such as Crohns, irritable bowel syndrome or ulcerative colitis, it may be necessary to use high doses over long periods. Always seek professional advice first.

Always take probiotics after a course of antibiotics. Do not take probiotics while you are still on antibiotics.

HOW TO SELECT THE RIGHT PROBIOTIC

The product should preferably be one that contains a multiculture of several bacteria, of which lactobacillus and bifidobacteria families are the most important. Other helpful species include streptococcus thermophilus and enterococcus faecium.

Refrigerated, freeze-dried products in powdered form are probably the best, although liquid mixed cultures are also acceptable. They have the advantage of containing beneficial bacterial metabolites that may have been lost during the process of freeze-drying.

Whatever form you choose, make sure that it is a high-potency product (containing at least two billion bacteria per capsule or dose), with stability data that indicate how the product will retain its potency. Check the expiry date.

High doses (five billion bacteria two to three times a day) are indicated after a course of antibiotics or to treat a specific condition where you have reason to believe that the gut microflora are involved. The best time to take the capsules is 20–30 minutes before a meal with a glass of water. This is to ensure the fastest passage of the bacteria through the harmful gastric acid environment in the stomach and destructive upper gastro-intestinal digestive juices. Before a meal, gastric acidity is low in the stomach.

For general prevention and maintenance, a dose of one billion bacteria three times a week is generally enough.

It's also a good idea to take supplements containing carbohydrate derivatives that will allow the administered bacteria to take hold and multiply faster. (Fructooligosaccharides – FOS – is widely used for this purpose. Take this preparation between meals as indicated on the package. Lactitol and sorbitol are other compounds that can be similarly used.)

CHAPTER EIGHT

MYTHS ABOUT MILK

Skilful advertising in the popular press over the years has given the impression that milk is the perfect food. Because of its high calcium content, it's an excellent way in which to build strong bodies in children and prevent osteoporosis in adults, we're told.

But is this so? To begin with, milk actually contains very little magnesium, yet magnesium is necessary to promote assimilation of calcium in the bones and prevent harmful deposition of calcium in the arterial walls and kidneys. (This deposition may promote the development of arterial atherosclerotic plaque).

Those who promote milk as a way of preventing osteoporosis have overlooked the fact that countries with the highest milk consumption are also those with the highest incidence of osteoporosis; Finland and Belgium have the highest milk consumption in Europe, as well as the highest incidence of osteoporosis, for example, although studies have not shown the role of risk factors (exercise, skin colour, physique) for osteoporosis in these examples.

Conversely, populations that consume little or no dairy products have the lowest incidence of osteoporosis, while animals other than humans that consume no milk do not have osteoporosis.

In evaluating the health aspects of milk, it is important to distinguish between what milk was 50–100 years ago, and what it is today. About a century ago, milk was consumed more or less straight from the cow. It was unpasteurised, unhomogenised and unpreserved, with all the beneficial enzymes intact. By the early 1900s, cows grazed free-range on natural pastures, consuming only natural grasses.

Today, throughout the world, cows are fed high-energy rations in sheds, with little or no opportunity for free-range grazing. This is, unfortunately, becoming increasingly common in South Africa as well.

In addition, cows have been selected to produce enormous, unphysiological quantities of milk every day; while two to four litres a day is normal, these animals are producing as much as 20 litres. It must be asked whether milk produced in such large quantities under artificial conditions is the same as the milk produced under more natural conditions.

Milk in the industrialised countries (including South Africa) today contains many foreign compounds, introduced largely as a result of agricultural practices.

These compounds include antibiotics and other drugs used to treat animals (some approved, some not); pesticides (reaching the animals via sprayed crops); bacteria from the pus of animals infected with heartwater and mastitis, which may include pathogens such as salmonella; genetically engineered growth hormones designed to increase milk production; and dangerous chemicals leached from plastic containers, which may include estrogens that have biological effects in minute quantities.

IMPORTANT DATES IN THE HISTORY OF MILK CONSUMPTION
➤ **Before 1900: The main fodder for cows was grass.**
➤ **1908: Pasteurisation, involving the heating of milk, was introduced to reduce spoilage and bacterial growth, at the same time altering the milk's protein structure and destroying beneficial enzymes.**
➤ **1919: Homogenisation of milk was introduced, which reduces the fat globules in milk into tiny particles that remain suspended and prevent the cream from separating.**
➤ **1932: Synthetic vitamin D was added to milk.**
➤ **1964: Plastic milk containers were commercially introduced to replace glass.**
➤ **1970: The use of antibiotics became widespread in animal feed, not only as treatment but to improve yield.**
➤ **1994: Genetically engineered growth hormone (also known as bovine growth hormone, or BGH) was introduced to further boost dairy yield per cow[243].**

THE BAD NEWS ABOUT MILK CONSUMPTION

In adults, the more full-cream milk you drink, the more likely it is that you may suffer from heart disease, arthritis, allergies, sinusitis, leukemia, lymphoma and other cancers, intestinal irritation and colic infections from salmonella.

Most of these diseases are linked to the foreign chemicals in milk that damage the immune system after chronic intake (around 500–1 000 ml a day, in the case of adults) of the contaminated milk. Thus the fat content of the milk does make a difference, as harmful chemicals are generally fat-soluble and accumulate in milk fat.

Despite what advertisers might say, milk is not a good source of minerals. Manganese, chromium, selenium and magnesium are found in higher concentrations in other foods, particularly vegetables, even if they're not organically grown.

Milk does indeed have a high calcium content, but a high intake of this food is likely to lead to a calcium-magnesium imbalance, with a relative magnesium deficiency. This may increase the risk of coronary heart disease, and has important implications for osteoporosis (see chapter two).

Many parents encourage their children to drink milk, so they will develop 'strong bones'. This results in the increased mucous production in their young children, as well as the increased incidence of a number of childhood diseases.

One of these is ear infection, which is becoming increasingly common[243]. Infection of the middle ear (otitis media) happens when ear secretions fail to drain properly and cause pressure, creating conditions that are favourable for infections.

Dairy products (excluding yoghurt and to a lesser extent cheese) are known to thicken secretions, making drainage from the blocked areas difficult. Antibiotics are usually the first line of treatment, yet seem to aggravate the situation.

A better approach is to avoid all dairy products and to keep the child well hydrated with copious quantities of water and herb teas. Unless the condition is serious, when antibiotics may have to be used, it is better to look to antimicrobial treatment with preparations such as golden leaf extract, which penetrates the mucous secretions.

Dairy products, and cow's milk in particular (even if it is organic and unpasteurised), have been implicated in a variety of other conditions, including eczema, fatigue, intestinal conditions, allergies, sinusitis, runny nose and childhood diabetes[243].

The high incidence of childhood diabetes in the dairy-consuming countries is revealing, as childhood type 1 (insulin dependent) diabetes has long been associated with a high intake of cow's milk (more than 50% of the daily caloric requirement) during the first months and possible first year of life. If an infant receives mother's milk for six months and gradually switches over to other foods, including perhaps some cow's milk, the effects are less serious.

Finland has, by far, the highest rate of type 1 diabetes (40/1 000 children) in children up to five years of age. In the United States, seven out of 1 000 children under the age of five have type 1 diabetes.

Studies have shown that diabetic children have levels of antibodies against milk protein (bovine serum albumin or BSA) eight times higher than healthy children[119]. There are at least 25 different proteins in cow's milk that can cause allergic reactions in humans, and the body may react to these as foreign invaders. These reactions may be responsible for the high incidence (75/1 000) of milk allergies in these children.

It may happen that the body, in an attempt to destroy the foreign invader by means of its own immune system, also damages some of its own tissues. Type 1 diabetes results from the destruction of the beta-cells in the pancreas by the immune system and is responsible for the deaths of 8 000 children a year in the UK alone.

ANOTHER REASON WHY BREAST IS BEST

Although not every mother is able to breast-feed, it is without doubt the case that mother's milk is the best food for a baby. Breast-fed infants have fewer and less severe illnesses, as well as fewer and less severe gastro-intestinal infections, respiratory and ear infections, eczema and asthma.

Breast milk promotes the growth of helpful intestinal bacteria that suppress the growth of disease-causing pathogens. Babies on milk-derived formulae have a level of healthy lactobacteria about 10% less than babies fed on mother's milk. (Soya milk formulae are better than cow's milk formulae, but not as good as breast-milk.)

And finally, some studies have shown that breast-fed babies score more highly on cognitive function tests than formula-fed babies. (These results do not necessarily include factors such as socio-economic status and the mother's education level, though.) Cow's milk was designed to meet the needs of the growing calf. One of these needs is the rapid development of muscles, hence its high protein and mineral content. A calf reaches a body weight of nearly 200 kg in six months, whereas a human infant grows only a few kilograms in six months.

On the other hand, rapid brain development is not a priority in calves, which is why cow's milk is much lower in essential fatty acids!

The human species has survived as a result of superior brain power, which is why mother's milk contains up to 10 times more essential fatty acids than that of cow's milk. One of these fatty acids is the vitally important omega-3 DHA (docosahexaenoic acid), an important component of brain cell membranes and the retina.

The omega-3 EPA (eicosapentaenoic acid) is another essential fatty acid that occurs in mother's milk, and its main function appears to be to fight infections.

The omega-6 fatty acid GLA (gamma linolenic acid), present in evening primrose oil, occurs in mother's milk, and this is our only dietary source of GLA. Although its specific function in infant nutrition is not clear, there is no doubt that it fulfills some essential function in the human infant. In infants and in adults, GLA plays an important function as the precursor of prostaglandin E1, which has a multitude of important functions (such as the regulation of nerve and metabolic functions in cells). GLA does not occur in cow's milk.

THE MAKING OF MILK

The milk we buy in stores has been pasteurised and homogenised, to make it safer and more convenient for human consumption.

During the process of pasteurisation, milk is subjected to elevated temperatures in order to reduce the count of harmful bacteria. At the same time, heat-sensitive vitamins such as vitamin D, necessary for the absorption of calcium, may be destroyed (although this is less of a problem in South Africa where were are exposed daily to vitamin-D rich sunlight). Raw milk also contains important enzymes that are necessary for the digestion of its proteins.

Population studies in Europe have implicated pasteurisation as a contributory cause of heart disease, although not the only factor. This is based on the sudden steep rise in heart disease seen in the UK and Norway within two years of the introduction of high-heat pasteurisation in 1931.

In the United States, deaths due to heart disease increased 12-fold between 1931–1945, when various heat processes were introduced in the manufacture of commercial milk and milk products. Although rapid urbanisation and the change to a diet high in refined foods played a role in this phenomenon, the sudden development of these conditions makes it more likely that heat treatment of milk was a contributory factor.

Among traditional Zulu people in South Africa, traditional Masai in Tanzania and Kenya, and nomadic peoples in Nigeria, milk is a key food, but it is consumed in the fermented form. The incidence of heart disease is very low in these peoples.

During the process of homogenisation, milk is subjected to intense agitation by means of which its fat droplets are broken up into tiny microdroplets. These microdroplets surround and entrap certain macromolecules, including the enzyme xanthine oxidase. This is an enzyme that contains the trace mineral molybdenum, which oxidises certain food components that also occur in DNA, including hypoxanthine, which is oxidised to the nitrogen-containing xanthine, and then to the nitrogen-containing uric acid.

Normally, in raw milk the enzyme is digested and does not enter the blood stream. However, in homogenised milk, the microdroplets entrap the enzyme and it is carried into the blood stream, where it produces a chemical that may damage the endothelium (innermost layer) in the artery walls. Quantities of as little as 500–1 000 ml of milk a day are enough to have this sort of impact on the body (the microdroplets that entrap the enzyme are absent from cheese and yoghurt).

Xanthine oxidase is known to destroy plasmologen, which makes up nearly 30% of the arterial wall cell membrane. This enzyme has been found in diseased sections of the heart and arterial wall in heart attack victims[121]. Through the deposition of calcium and cholesterol, plaque starts to form – the beginning of the process of atherosclerosis.

Groups of people who consume no milk products are free from plaque formation and atherosclerotic heart disease. On the other hand, in experimental animals, cats fed homogenised milk suffered rapid and profound degeneration[122].

Some experts such as Dr K Oster, former head of cardiology at Chicago hospital, believes that up to 50% of all heart disease is initiated through xanthine oxidase entering the circulation in this manner.

WHAT ELSE IS IN THE MILK WE DRINK?

During the last 20 years, 6 000 chemicals have been introduced into our food and the world around us, while 40% of pesticides have been shown to be toxic to the nervous system as well as carcinogenic and mutagenic (able to cause abnormalities in the genetic material during cellular replication). Many other pesticides are known to have estrogenic activity, adding to the estrogen load to which we are exposed. Others, like the organic chemicals in plastic, are able to mimic the effect of natural estrogens.

In 1996, there were three million cases of severe pesticide poisoning, and 20 000 deaths could be attributed to pesticides.

Most of these toxins are predominantly fat-soluble, and when they enter the body they tend to concentrate in body fats. In cows, this means the fats in milk.

The antibiotics in milk also pose a big health problem. Information obtained from the Consumer Union in the US indicate that the meat and dairy industries are the biggest users of antibiotics. These are added to feed to improve animal growth and for the treatment of a variety of animal diseases; 52 drugs are used to treat mastitis alone. These drugs and their metabolites go directly into the animals' milk, and the required withdrawal time after drug treatment (up to seven milking periods or 70 litres of milk) are seldom observed, for obvious financial reasons.

Moreover, for some drugs, approval times have not yet been established, with the result that nobody knows when the milk of cows treated in this manner is safe for human consumption. The result is that in the US, at least, about 30% of all commercial milk products are contaminated with antibiotic residues.

These drugs, even at low levels, are capable of inducing allergic reactions in a certain small percentage of consumers. Milk is the most common dietary item involved in food allergies, and both the milk proteins as well as the antibiotic and drug residues in the milk may be the cause.

Constantly ingesting small amounts of antibiotics may also have other serious health effects, some of which are not directly noticeable by the consumer. These residues may create favourable conditions for the development of resistant strains of bacteria, which may have serious long-term consequences for us all.

Perhaps even more importantly, these antibiotics tend to upset the delicate and all-important intestinal bacteria in the consumer (see chapter seven).

A weak immune system (eg frequent colds) can frequently be linked to an imbalanced gut flora brought about by the presence of antibiotic residues in milk even though the patient may not have received antibiotic treatment recently.

WHAT ABOUT CHEESE?

If raw milk is contaminated with antibiotics and other chemicals to the extent shown above, products derived from such milk are likely to be contaminated too. Cheese and butter are concentrated forms of milk, and the concentration of contaminants will be accordingly higher.

At least 21 kg of milk is necessary to produce 1 kg of butter or 2 kg of cheese, while 11 kg of milk is necessary to produce 1 kg of non-fat dried milk powder. Fortunately the actual amount of these toxins you ingest will be offset by the fact that you eat proportionately less of these products than when you drink milk.

The average milk consumer will drink about 400 ml of milk a day, but eat only around 50 g of cheese. The annual intake per person of milk products in America is more than 400 kg per year (40% of the American diet). In addition to the milk products mentioned, there are a multitude of other foods that contain hidden dairy products in the form of milk powder, cream and ice cream. There are a growing number of Americans who are now avoiding milk but these hidden sources of milk products are difficult to avoid.

LACTOSE INTOLERANCE

Lactose is the primary sugar in cow and mother's milk. Infants produce the enzyme lactase, which is needed to digest lactose. Genetic factors are responsible for the fact that after weaning, many people can no longer produce the enzyme, indicating that milk is not intended as a food for adults.

People who cannot produce lactase can develop mild to serious problems, depending on whether no lactase at all is produced or whether its level of production is inadequate. The usual symptoms include diarrhoea, bloating, gas, cramps and allergies.

The genetic feature to stop lactase production after weaning is common, and it occurs in many different races. Therefore lactose intolerance in an individual should not be considered a disease. Many northern Europeans, perhaps as a result of the centuries' old tradition of milk consumption, are capable of tolerating lactose, while among black South Africans, for example, lactose intolerance is widespread.

LIVING WITHOUT MILK

Most people will find it very difficult to avoid milk and milk products entirely, but by limiting consumption to one or two cups a day and by selecting fat-free and organically produced milk, the possible damage can be limited. What is wrong is to consume large quantities (one or more litres a day) in an attempt to prevent osteoporosis (see chapter two).

If you crave the taste and feel of dairy, or when recipes require cream or milk, consider substituting with yoghurt or soya milk (if you do not suffer from thyroid problems).

CHAPTER NINE

THE MASS APPEAL
OF MARGARINE

Margarine was developed in the mid-1900s to make available, on a massive scale, a cheap source of polyunsaturated fats (PUFAs) that could be used as a spread to compete with butter; and to find a profitable outlet for large quantities of the newly available polyunsaturated marine and plant oils.

Saturated fats (such as those found in butter) were regarded as an important cause of heart disease because of their association with raised blood cholesterol values (see chapter one).

So, when it was discovered that the partial catalytic hydrogenation of marine and plant oils could convert them into semi-solid products with much the same properties as butter, two problems seemed to have been simultaneously solved: the control of cholesterol levels by means of dietary polyunsaturated fats; and provision of a ready outlet for the polyunsaturated oils (see chapter one).

When clinical studies showed that inclusion of the newly developed margarine did indeed lower blood cholesterol levels somewhat, the headlong rush to popularise margarine as the solution to heart problems was on!

The idea that cholesterol-lowering was the solution to heart problems was so entrenched in the mid-1900s that it was not considered necessary to run trials to see whether margarine consumption actually reduced heart attack incidence and death rate.

No follow-up studies were conducted where heart attack incidence was monitored among a group of margarine consumers and a group of butter consumers, for example.

And when eventually trials were done (in the 1970s) and the results were not quite as expected, the whole matter was swept under the carpet with the help of virtually unlimited advertising and research funds from the food industry.

Generations have grown up believing that margarine (also called hydrogenated vegetable oil) is a superior 'health' food, the longed-for answer to many health problems.

HOW IS MARGARINE PRODUCED?

The chemical composition of oils and fats is a combination of the alcohol glycerol combined with long-chain fatty acids, often the type of fatty acid that contains 18 carbon atoms joined together in a row.

Hard fats such as lard contain mostly saturated fatty acids, which means that all the positions on the carbon atoms have been taken up by hydrogen atoms, leaving no 'vacancies'. When two hydrogen molecules have been removed from two adjacent carbon molecules in the fatty acid chain, the bonds that come free are joined so as to form a second carbon-carbon bond. This is called a 'double bond', and because it represents a site of increased chemical activity, it is called 'unsaturated'.

When several such double bonds occur in the same molecule, the molecule is called 'polyunsaturated'.

Saturated fatty acids consist of long carbon chains joined together by single bonds.

Liquid oils are made up predominantly of unsaturated fatty acid oils, in which one or more 'vacancies' (double bonds) exist. These vacancies can take up hydrogen atoms and therefore become solid fats – this process is called 'hydrogenation', and in order to speed up the process, chemists can carry out the reaction at high temperatures in the presence of a catalyst such as platinum. The process is then called 'catalytic hydrogenation'.

The vacancies on the molecule that can take up additional hydrogens in this manner are called 'double bonds'.

A monounsaturated fatty acid has one double bond (such as in olive oil), and a polyunsaturated fatty acid has two double bonds (such as in sunflower oil).

The more double bonds a molecule has, the more fluid the product tends to be and vice versa. Thus, by reducing the number of double bonds in a molecule through the process of catalytic hydrogenation, the product tends to become more solid, like butter.

In addition, they disrupt the vital functions of essential fatty acids by interfering with the enzymes that transform these into prostaglandins, which are vital for normal cellular functions and therefore health.

Trans fatty acids also have many other harmful effects at the enzyme level by interfering with the detoxification of chemical insecticides and enhancing other insecticides that have the ability to make carcinogens more potent.

WHERE DO WE FIND TRANS FATTY ACIDS?

The percentage of trans fatty acids in margarines vary, from approximately 15–26% in tub margarines and 40–50% in block margarines.

About 95% of the average intake of trans fatty acids comes from hydrogenated vegetable oils in the form of margarines (a mixture of cis and trans fatty acids), other shortenings and oils.

Other trans fatty acids in our diet come from animal products such as beef (up to 10%) and butter (up to 9%) – this is because trans fatty acids are produced in the rumen of cattle fed on high-energy grain concentrates. Venison is very low in trans fatty acids, as game don't eat grain concentrates; mutton may also be low in trans fatty acids, particularly if the animals grazed on natural pastures.

THE MASS MARKET FOR MARGARINE

Margarine has found its way into thousands of sweet and savoury products on our food shelves. Bread, rolls, pies, pastries, biscuits, cakes, muffins, hamburgers, potato chips, salad dressings, mayonnaise and peanut butter are just a few examples among hundreds of other products.

Dietary surveys indicate that the average per capita intake of trans fatty acids in the United States is 8 g per day, which translates into 20–30 g of hydrogenated oil per day (approximately 16–25 ml a day).

In the US there have been organised campaigns, for example by the Heartsavers Foundation, to persuade consumers to eat hydrogenated vegetable oils, while the fast food chain McDonalds has announced with great fanfare that they will use 'vegetable oil' rather than beef tallow to fry their French fries.

However, the beef tallow used at present is lower in fatty acid content than margarine! Moreover, the term 'hydrogenated vegetable oil' is misleading as it creates the impression that pure plant oils are to be used. In fact, companies have not switched to pure vegetable oils, but rather to shortenings produced from hydrogenated vegetable oils. Beef tallow contains about 4% trans fatty acids, while hydrogenated soya oil contains 42%.

According to the FDA in the US, seven out of eight packaged foods contain trans fats. The labels on such products claim that they are 'low in saturated fats', which is literally true, but which omits the fact that from a health point of view, they are worse than the animal fats they have been produced to replace.

The campaign to switch from animal fats to margarines has not only been widely promoted by food companies but has also received enthusiastic support from the medical profession and dietetic associations (see chapter one).

The situation in South Africa has been no different to that in the United States. During the increase in heart attack incidence in the 1960s, the medical profession and the Heart Foundation strongly promoted the use of hydrogenated oils and margarines, with glossy print and television advertising as well as high-profile public awareness campaigns.

This support has persisted, despite scientific evidence that these products are not only unhealthy but that they may actually cause heart attacks (see below).

WHAT'S THE EVIDENCE?

First indications that margarine may not be a healthy alternative to animal fats came from animal experiments in the 1950s.

Experiments on pigs fed a basic diet to which different types of fat (beef tallow, butter, egg yolk powder, crystalline cholesterol and hydrogenated oil) were added showed that the hydrogenated vegetable oil group had the most atherosclerosis with lesions in the aortas.

As early as 1956, there were already indications of the harmful effects in humans. In 1956, the editor of the *Lancet* stated that 'coronary artery disease becomes in part a preventable disorder, but at the cost of a complete revolution of our present day dietary habits. The hydrogenation plants of our modern food industry may turn out to have contributed to the causation of a major disease.'

This was followed by an increasing number of human studies, all with bad news for the margarine supporters. In 1997 a study showed that women with the highest level of trans fat stores in their tissues had a 40% increased risk of developing breast cancer than those with the lowest levels[82]. Trans fats raise the levels of triglycerides and of Lipoprotein a, both known risk factors for heart disease.

A study published in the *Lancet* by the Harvard School of Medicine showed that trans fatty acids increase concentrations of LDL ('bad' cholesterol), while at the same time decreasing the levels of the HDL ('good' cholesterol). Both of these effects may be expected to increase the heart disease risk[83].

In another study, published in 1993 in the *Lancet*, 85 095 women (no history of stroke or heart disease or raised cholesterol) were studied for a period of eight years. After adjustment for age, energy intake, other risk factors for heart disease, vitamin use etc, the results showed that the group with the highest intake of margarine had a relative risk of 1,5 compared to 1 for the group with the lowest intake. In other words, the high margarine group had a 50% increased risk for heart attacks.

A similar study (*Lancet* 1992) showed that regular consumption of margarine increases the risk for heart disease significantly. There was a greatly increased risk when daily margarine consumption increased to 20 g (five teaspoons, or 25 ml). Cakes and other cereal products prepared with margarine also increase the risk.

A further study done in 1997 found that while margarine intake increases heart risk, butter does not[84].

The definitive study, published in the *Lancet*, came in 2001[85]. In this eight-year study on 85 000 nurses, it was found that those with the highest intake of hydrogenated vegetable oil (margarine) had the highest rate of heart disease.

These studies enjoyed widespread interest in the non-scientific and popular media, with headlines such as 'Epidemiologists link margarine to heart attacks' (*Food Chemical News*, 29 March 1993); 'Study links heart disease to margarine' (*New York Times*, 5 March 1993); and 'US study says margarine may be harmful' (*New York Times*, 7 October 1992).

Ironically, these studies showed that the very condition they were introduced to prevent – heart disease – is actually aggravated by their use.

Technically, trans fats are unsaturated and thus classified by many as 'polyunsaturated fats', the one-time darling of cardiologists. Metabolically, they resemble saturated fats more closely, but they are more harmful than these fats in more than one way.

MAKING DECISIONS ABOUT FATS

Although warnings that margarine and hydrogenated fats may be harmful to health and that they may increase the risk of heart attacks, some medical doctors and dieticians have continued to promote the use of these products. This is partly due to a medical preoccupation with cholesterol as the principal cause of heart disease, and partly as a result of advertising pressure to boost margarine sales based on medical endorsement.

What should you do in the face of such advice from health-care professionals?

A good start is to be as fully informed as possible. And having carefully considered the above evidence, the basic problem to solve is, which fats are good and which ones are bad?

If the choice is between butter and margarine, clearly butter is the victor.

However, before you rejoice in the thought of endless feasts of rich foods, remember that too much butter may also not be a good thing.

Firstly, some of the hormones and artificial chemicals used in agricultural practice accumulate in body fat, and in this manner may land on your table (see page 132). Try to find butter produced from cows that have not been treated with production-boosting hormones.

For all cooking and salad-dressing purposes, use virgin, cold-pressed olive oil. I use a 50:50 mix of olive oil and butter as a spread. It tastes good and does not become hard in the fridge, plus it's an easy way to prevent excessive intake of butter. For baking, use canola or light olive oil – ask at a local Italian delicatessen for this product. Avoid commercial cooking oils such as sunflower oil; these oils have been chemically treated.

Sesame oil and peanut oil are good, provided they were produced organically, while coconut milk is good in moderate quantities.

Never eat food that has been prepared in overheated vegetable oil; these oils are easily oxidised on heating, and when they have been used repeatedly they are especially bad, so this means, effectively, no commercially prepared potato chips!

It is acceptable to use essential fatty acid supplements containing cod liver oil, flaxseed oil, fish oil and evening primrose oil, but take care to store them in well-closed dark bottles away from sunshine and in the refrigerator. Expose these oils as little as possible to air and only open them for the daily dose.

CHAPTER TEN

SOURCES OF NUTRIENTS

There is an ever-increasing awareness of the importance of nutrition, especially of micronutrients, among medical professionals and the general public. This has created a growing market for products containing them, which in turn has attracted the attention of large numbers of manufacturers. Unfortunately, some manufacturers market inferior products, often promoted by excessive and irresponsible claims.

Reputable manufacturers and companies may be recognised by the fact that they offer substantial documentation, backed by scientific references, on which their products are based. Quality products are identifiable by applying the following criteria:

➤ Products must contain significant quantities of vitamins and minerals – the amounts must at least be RDA related. For instance, a product that contains 10 mg of magnesium per daily dose is meaningless because the RDA for magnesium is 400 mg.

➤ In the case of minerals, make sure that the quantities listed on the label refer to the elemental content. For example, a product that lists magnesium chloride (550 mg) as one of its ingredients, in fact contains only 65 mg of elemental magnesium since the salt 'magnesium chloride' contains only 11,96% of elemental magnesium.

➤ In the majority of cases, it is not advisable to take nutrients in isolation, ie on their own, because of the principle of synergism. For example, magnesium must be taken in combination with zinc, manganese and copper, and individual B vitamins are best taken in the form of a multivitamin. Calcium should not be taken alone, for example, for the treatment of osteoporosis, but preferably with adequate quantities of magnesium and other minerals.

➤ Most micronutrients, especially the water-soluble B vitamins, are best taken in slow-release form to mimic the way in which food naturally delivers these nutrients to the body.

Most health shops and pharmacies stock a wide range of products. Unusual supplements such as acetylcarnitine for sufferers of Alzheimer's disease, which are not readily available, are also obtainable on a 24-hour mail order basis. These supplements, as well as a series of information files on selected diseases such as cancer and heart disease, are obtainable from Fortifood Health Services (Pty) Ltd, PO Box 26447, Monument Park, Pretoria 0105, tel: (012) 3461703, fax: (012) 3462206, e-mail: Fortifood@worldonline.co.za

REFERENCES

1   *New England Journal of Medicine* 2002; 347: 81

2   *JAMA* 2002; 288: 321

3   *JAMA* 2000; 284: 483

4   *JAMA* 1994; 272: 1851

5   *JAMA* 1998; 279: 1200

6   Serfontein WJ. *New Nutrition.* Cape Town: Tafelberg Publishers; 2002

7   *Am J Med Sc* 1990; 299: 207

8   *Age and Aging* 1999; 28: 313

9   *JAMA* 1991; 266: 1225

10 *Virchows Arch Pathol Anat Histopath* 1990; 417(2): 105

11 *Circulation* Sept 2000

12 *Life Extension Foundation Treatment Protocols: Fibronogen and Cardiovascular disease*

13 *Lancet* 17 Jan 1987; 155

14 *BMJ* 8 April 1989; 920

15 *Arch Int Med* 1992; 152: 1371

16 *Lancet* 1925; 1: 1270

17 *Medical History* 1985; suppl. no 5: 141

18   *J Royal Coll Gen Practitioners* April 1987; 174

19   Serfontein WJ. *Hidden Health Hazards.* Cape Town: Tafelberg Publishers; 2003

20   *Lancet* 11 Aug 1873; 298

21   *Lancet* 20 June 1992; 1423

22   *Lancet* 19 March 1977; 654

23   *American Heart Association Monograph No 25*; 1969

24   *Townsend Letter* April 2001; 76

25   *Cancer Research Institute Monograph No 18* (on breast cancer) 1984; 91

26   *JAMA* 1966; 129

27   *Circulation* March1968

28   *Lancet* 1971; 464

29   *World Review of Nutr Dietetics* 1970; 12: 1–42

30   *Transact Am Clin Climatol Assoc* 1973; 85: 100

31   *Am J Clin Nutr* May 1967; 462

32   *Lancet* 14 Nov 1987; 1144

33   *Int Surg* 1991; 76: 1

34   *Artery* 1979; 5: 170

35   *Proc Natl Acad Sc* 1991; 88: 1646

36   *J Cardiovasc Res* 1996; 3: 352

37   *Eur Heart J* 2000; 21: 1591

38   *J Lipid Res* 2000; 41: 1552

39   *Cardiovasc Drugs Ther* 2000; 4: 397

40   *Cerebrovasc Dis* 2001; 11 (1): 85

41   *JAMA* 1991; 266: 1225

42   *BMJ* 1984; 288: 424

43   *Lancet* 1994; 344: 1383

44   *Lancet* 1996; p 781

45   Serfontein WJ. *Beating Cancer.* Cape Town: Tafelberg; 2002

46   *JAMA* 1995; 275: 55

47   *Proc Natl Acad Sc* 1990; 87: 8931

48   *Nature Medicine* 2000; 6: 1311

49   *Virchows Arch Pathol Anat Histopath* 1990; 417 (2): 105

50   *J Opt Nutr* 3 Nov 1993:

51   *Neurol Teratol* 1995; 17: 31

52   *Int J Clin Pharm Res* 1999; XIX (4):117

53   *J Pharm Pharmacol* 1995; 47: 289

54   *Physiol Behav* 1999; 67: 1

55   *Pharmacol Res* 1997; 36: 293

56   *Int J Clin Pharmacol Therap* 1998; 36: 469

57   *Curr Therap Res* 1997; 58: 390

58   Pauling Linus. *How to live longer and feel better.* Avon Books; 1986

59   *Canad Med Ass J* 1957; 77: 15

60   *Proc Natl Acad Sc USA* 1990; 87: 9388 (Bioch)

61   *Europ Heart J* 1990; Suppl. E: 174

62   *New Engl J Med* 1990; 322: 1494

63   *J Orthomol Med* 1991; 6: 144

64   *J Am Coll Cardiol* 1998; 41: 980

65   *Epidemiology* 1992; 3: 194

66   *BMJ* 1997; 314 (7081): 634

67   *Lancet* 2001; 357 (9257): 657

68   *JAMA* 2002; 288: 3

69   *JAMA* 1998; 280: 605

70   *JAMA* 2000; 283: 1007

71   *New Engl J Med* 1989; 321: 293

72   *Lancet ii* 1979; 33

73   *New Engl J Med* 1993; 329: 114

74   *Am J Med* 1988; 85: 847

75   *JAMA* 2002; 287: 734

76   Colgan M. *Hormonal Health.* Vancouver: Apple Publishing; 1996

77   *Townsend Letter* Feb/March 2002; p 115

78   *Townsend Letter* Feb/March 2002; p 166

79   *Townsend Letter* Feb/March 2002; p 150

80   *Horm Metab Res* 1987; 19: 579

81   *Zentrbl Gynakol* 1988; 110: 611

82   *Am J Clin Nutr* 1997; 66s (1): 1548s

83   *Am J Clin Nutr* 1997; 66s (1): 1006s

84   *Epidemiology* 1997; 8: 144

85   *Lancet* 2001; 357: 746

86   *Calcif Tiss Intern* 1987; 41: 57

87   *Am J Clin Nutr* 1988; 48: 712

88   *J Nutr Med* 1991; 2: 167

89   *J Royl Soc Med* 1994; 87 (27): 27

90   *BMJ* 1990; 300: 1056

91   *BMJ* 1989; 298: 137

92   *Calcified Tiss Intern* 1990;46: 300

93   *J Nutr Med* 1991; 2: 168

94   *Scand J Clin Lab Invest* 1958; 10: 36

95   *Min Electrol Metab* 1993;19: 314

96   *J Am Coll Nutr* 1993; 12: 601

97   *Magn Bull* 1989; 4: 3

98   *Magn Bull* 189; 4: 5

99   *Am J Clin Nutr* 1999; 69: 727

100   *J Nutr Med* 1991; 2: 170

101   *J Nutr Med* 1991; 2: 165

102   Serfontein W J. *New Nutrition.* Cape Town: Tafelberg Publishers; 1991

103   *Magn Res* 1989; 2: 142

104   *Calcif Tiss Res* 1972; 10:269

105   *J Nutr* 1996; 126 (14): 1187s

106   *Metabolism* 1998; 47: 195

107   *Endocrinology* 1998; 139: 10

108   *Am J Clin Nutr* 1993; 12: 384

109   *Environm Health Perspectives* 1994; 102 (7): 83

110   *J Biol Chem* 1984; 259: 5403

111   Lee JR. *Natural Progesterone.* United Kingdom: Jon Carpenter Publishing; 1996

112   *Intern Clin Nutr Rev* 1990; 10: 384

113   *Biochemical Med* 1972; 6: 526

114   *Metabolism* 1985; 11: 1073

115   *Townsend Letter* Oct 2002; 128

116   Cohen R. *Milk: the Deadly Poison.* New Jersey: Argus Publ; 1998

117   Miami Dade. *Natural Healing: Relief for Ear Infections.* June 2002

118   *Health and Healing* 1996; 6: 106

119   *The Immuno Rev* 1994; 2:3

120   Brown H, *et al. The Key to Ultimate Health.* California: Advanced Health Research; 2000

121   Oster, K A, Ross D J, *et al. The XO factor: and How It Can Destroy Your Arteries, Your Heart, Your Life!* New York, Park City Press; 1983

122   *Health Science Institute* Nov 2002

123   *New Engl J Med* 2001; Oct 25: 1230

124   *Cancer* 2001; 91: 2214

125   *Acta Physiol Scand* 1987; 129: 47

126   Colgan M. *Optimum Sports Nutrition.* New York: Advanced Research Press; 1993

127   *J Am Acad Dermatol* 19 Oct (4): 642

128   *Rev Med Intern* 2000; 21: 946; *Ann Rev Nutr* 1999; 19: 357; *Tidskr Nor Laegefor* 1990; 110

129   *Ann Nutr Metab* 1997; 41: 203

130   *New Engl J Med* 25 Oct 2001; 1230

131   *Cancer* 2001; 91: 2214

132   *J Am Geriatr Soc* 2001; 49: 1226

133   Emory T. *Iron and Your Health: Facts and Fallacies.* CRC; 1991

134   *Science* 1975; 188: 1038

135   Bullen DJ, Griffiths E. *Iron and Infection.* New York: John Wiley; 1987

136   *New Engl J Med* April1994; 1152

137   *Am Coll Gyn Obstr* Sept 1987; 1

138   *Circulation* 1992; 86: 803

139   *Can J Psych* 1994; 39: 8

140   *JAMA* 26 March 1997

141   Zilva J, Panall PR. *Clinical Chemistry in Diagnosis and Treatment.* London: Lloyd–Luke; 1984

142   *Am J Clin Nutr* 2001; 73: 152,155

143   *J Pediatr* 1999; 135: 564

144   Nurition Sc News Dec 2000

145   *Lancet* 2001; 357: 1076

146   *J Am Dietet Assoc* 2001; 101: 229

147   *J Appl Nutr* 36: 125

148   Rasic J. *Bifido Bacteria and their Role.* Boston: Birkhauser Verlag; 1983

149   *Gut* 13: 251

150   *See* text books on immunology.

151   *SA J Nat Med* 2001; 2: 38

152   *New Scientist* 18 July 1992; 31

153   *Science* 1999; 286: 1353

154   Shilts R. *And the Band Played On: Politics, People and the AIDS Epidemic.* New York: St. Martin's Press; 1988

155   *Nature* 2000; vol 406

156   *Science* 1999; 286: 1353

157   Foster Harold D. *What Really Causes AIDS.* Trafford Publishing; 2002

158   *UNAIDS/WHO Epidemiological Fact Sheet on HIV/AIDS* 2000; Uganda: update (revised)

159   *UNAIDS/WHO Epidemiological Fact Sheet on HIV/AIDS* 2000; S Africa: update (revised)

160   *UNAIDS/WHO Epidemiological Fact Sheet on HIV/AIDS* 2000; Senegal: update (revised)

161   Hecht D. *AIDS Among Senegalese Sex Workers Inexplicably Low.* April 1997; *Drum:* 5

162   *UNAIDS/WHO Epidemiological Fact Sheet on HIV/AIDS* 2000; S Africa: update (revised)

163   *AIDS* 1999; 13: 1397

164   *J Acquired Imm Def Syndr and Human Retrovirology* 1997; 15: 370

165   *The Lancet* 2001; 357: 1651

166   *Cancer* 1996; 77: 2132

167   *Nature* 2000; 406

168   *Science* 2000; 287: 607

169   *Cancer* 1996; 77: 2132

170   *New Scientist* July 18 July 1992; 32

171   *Proc Natl Acad Sc* 1997

172   *Fed Proc Am Soc Exp Biol* 1982; 41: 3570

173   *J Immunol* 1985; 135: 2740

174   *Immunol Today* 1994; 15: 7

175   *Proc Natl Acad Sc USA* 1997; 94: 1967

176   *Nutrition* 1999; 15: 165

177   *AIDS Res Human Retrovir* 1994

178   *J Orthomol Med* 1997; 12: 227

179   Howe GM. *International Variations in Cancer Incidence and Mortality.*
       Edinburgh: Churchill Livingstone; 1986: 3–42

180   *Geochim Cosmochim Acta* 1966; 30: 769

181   Furon R. *The Problem of Water.* London: Faber and Faber; 1967

182   Oldfield JE. *Selenium World Atlas.* Grimbergen, Belgium: Selenium-Tellurium
       Development Association; 1999

183   Editorial Board. *The Atlas of Endemic Diseases and the Environments in the
       People's Republic of China.* Beijing: Science Press; 1985

184   *Biol Trace Elem Res* 1999; 70: 97

185   *Intern Symp on Environm Life Elements and Health* 1–5 Nov 1988; p 241: Beijing

186   *Biol Trace Elem Res* 1997; 56: 31

187   *Z Ernahrungswiss* 1988; 37 (1): 118

188   *Townsend Letter* April 2002; 76

189   *Nutrition* 1999; 15: 860

190   *J Interferon Res* 1990; 10: 599

191   *Biochem Bioph Res Comms* 1995; 207: 258

192   *Q J Exp Physiol* 1985; 70: 473

193   *Ann Surg* 1994; 226: 212

194   *Med Hyp* 1996; 46: 252

195   *Nutrition* 1999; 15: A 68

196   *Blood* 1998; 91: 3817

197   *Bioch Bioph Res Comms* 1988; 153: 888

198   *New Eng J Med* 1998; 338: 853

199   Garrett L. *The Betrayal of Trust: the Collapse of Global Public Health.* New York:
       Hyperion; 2000

200   *Nature* 2000; vol 406

201   Hooper E. *The River: A Journey to the Source of HIV and AIDS.* Boston:
       Little Brown; 1999

202   *Virus Genes* 2001; 23: 215

203   *New Scientist* 19 Sept 1992; 8

204   Yang GQ, *et al. Selenium in Biology and Medicine.* New York: Van Nostrand
       Reinhold Company; 1987; pp 589, 859

205   *Biol Trace Elem Res* 1989; 20: 15

206   *University of Cambridge Cancer Intelligence Unit Report*; June1997

207   Abel U. *Chemotherapy of Advanced Epithelial Cancer: A Critical Survey.* Stutgart: Hippokrates Verlag; 1990

208   Bjorksten. *Longevity.* Charlston: JAB Publications; 1987; p 22.

209   *Univ of Cambridge Cancer Intelligence Unit Report* June 1997

210   *New England J Med* 1984; 310: pp 633, 697

211   Moss R. *Questioning Chemotherapy.* New York: Equinox Press; 2000

212   Braverman A. *Lancet* 1991; 337: 901

213   *Brit J Cancer* 1986; 54: 661

214   *J Clin Oncol* 1987; 5: 1711

215   *Proc ASCO(Abstract No 455)* 1988; 7: 118

216   Jonssen B, Karlsson G. *Introducing New Treatments for Cancer: Economic Evaluation of Cancer Treatments.* In: Williams CJ, editor. New York: John Wiley; 1992

217   *Science* 1995; 267: 1047

218   *Science Writers* 1994–1995; 42: 14

219   Abel U. *Chemotherapy of Advanced Epithelial Cancer: A Critical Survey.* Stutgart: Hippokrates Verlag; 1990

220   Zinner NR. Prostate. In: Dollinger M, *et al. Everyone's Guide to Cancer Therapy.* Toronto: Somerville House Books; 1991; 485

221   *New Engl J Med* 1994; 331: 810

222   *Proc Am Ass Canc Res* 1982; 23: 155

223   *Chest* 1991; 99: 1325

224   Pauling L. *How to Live Longer and Feel Better.* New York: WH Freeman; 1986

225   *Postgrad Med* 1990; 87: 163

226   *Am J Clin Nutr* 1991; 53: 270s

227   Simone CB. *Cancer and Nutrition: A Ten-Point Plan to Reduce your Risk of Getting Cancer.* New York: Avery Publishing Group Inc.; 1994

228   *CA Cancer J Clin* 1992; 42: 181

229   Cameron E, Pauling L. *Cancer and Vitamin C.* Philadelphia: Camino Books; 1993

230   *B Bull Surg Res* 2002; 3: 278

231   *Arch Int Med* 1982; 142: 42

When a fluid polyunsaturated oil such as soya oil is subject to controlled catalytic hydrogenation, the process may be intercepted at a stage before all the double bonds have been saturated, and it is thus semi-solid.

Margarine is produced in this way, and because the product on average still contains more than one double bond per molecule, it is defined as 'polyunsaturated'.

THE CONSEQUENCES OF TRANS FATTY ACIDS

The molecular configuration of natural fatty acids is called a 'cis configuration' where both of the remaining two hydrogen atoms on the double bond (see opposite) lie on the same side.

When subject to high temperatures, as in catalytic hydrogenation or during high temperature cooking, the molecule of a natural fatty acid 'flips over' or twists, so the two hydrogen atoms lie on opposite sides of the double bond. This is called a 'trans configuration' (as opposed to a cis configuration), and the resulting product is called a trans fatty acid.

The result of such a change is far reaching in biological terms. The trans fatty acid molecule now no longer fits into sites on the cellular membranes and enzymes where the cis form of the molecule would fit. This is because structurally the two types of fatty acids take up different 'shapes' of space on the chain, so do not fit on the same site on the membrane.

A trans fatty acid molecule is therefore not able to perform the natural functions of the cis form, as structural components of cell membranes and as precursors of cellular messengers. Worse still, a trans fatty acid may compete with the natural form, thus blocking it out from vital processes.

In this manner the trans fatty acids in margarine have many harmful effects. No matter how little of the product you eat, these trans fats contribute to the increased stickiness of the fatty acid molecule, which then encourages fatty deposits in the artery walls. They also increase the stickiness of blood platelets, thus increasing the likelihood of the formation of a blood clot, especially in the smaller blood vessels, leading to strokes and heart attacks.

Furthermore, by being incorporated at the sites normally occupied by the cis molecules, they alter the permeability of cell membranes, allowing entry into the cell of undesirable molecules that are ordinarily kept out of a cell, and they also allow vital molecules in the cell to escape.

232   *J Clin Pharmacol* 1998; 38: 792

233   Serfontein WJ. *New Nutrition.* Cape Town: Tafelberg Publishers; 2001

234   *JAMA* 2000; 283:1007

235   *New Engl J Med 1993; 329: 114*

236   JAMA 2002; 287: 734

237   *Townsend Letter* March 2002; 116

238   *JAMA* 1998; 280: 605

239   *New Engl J Med* 1990; 322: 1–6

240   *Townsend Letter* Nov 2003; 110

241   *SAJ Nat Med* 2001; 5: 66

242   *SAJ Nat Med* 2001; 2: 38

243   *Townsend Letter* Oct 2002; 128, Nov 2002; 48

.

INDEX

3TC *see* antiretrovirals

acquired immune deficiency syndrome *see* AIDS

AIDS 79–101 *see also* HIV
    causes 80, 82
    diagnostic diseases 80, 82, 85, 90
    Durban declaration 82
    Incidence 79, 85
    mortality 79, 82, 86, 90, 91, 97
    nutrient deficiencies 83, 88, 93, 99–100

alcohol 49, 109, 124, 128

allergies 124, 127, 128, 133, 134, 136, 138

anaemia 69–76
    in elderly 69, 70, 71, 72, 73–74

tests for 70

antibiotics 123, 124, 126, 128, 129, 132, 133, 136

antioxidants 13–14, 15, 16, 17, 18, 24, 26, 28, 35, 63, 64, 83, 88, 89, 95, 116, 117

antiretrovirals (ARVs) 79, 80, 81, 82, 95, 98

apoptosis 95

aromatase 71

arteries 11, 14, 15, 17, 32, 34, 44, 45, 143
    plaques 11, 14, 17, 26, 32, 33–34, 131

arteriosclerosis 44

atherosclerosis 17, 24, 25, 30, 32, 34, 44, 131, 136, 145

AZT *see* antiretrovirals

B

B-lymphocytes *see* lymphocytes
bacteria 74, 81, 123, 124, 125, 126, 132, 135, 136
  beneficial *see* probiotics
bifidobacteria 124, 128, 129
bioflavonoids 17
Black Cohosh 65–66
blood
  clotting 11, 29, 30, 32, 36, 45, 55, 61, 64, 143 *see also* warfarin
  fats *see* triglycerides
  ferritin 69
bone 41, 43, 44, 45, 46, 47, 60, 133
  fractures 39, 40, 41, 44, 45, 49, 55
  fragility 39, 44, 45, 55
  loss 40, 41, 43, 46, 47, 48–49, 60
  scans 48
boron 43, 46, 49
bovine growth hormone (BGH) 132, 147
breast-feeding
  and HIV 86
breast milk 74, 124, 133–135, 138
  see also milk
butter 16, 18–19, 21, 22-23, 136, 141, 142, 145, 146, 147 *see also* saturated fats

C

C-reactive protein (CPR) 36
CAD *see* coronary artery disease
calcification 44 *see also* arteries
calcium 39–43, 44, 45, 48, 49, 85, 131, 133, 135, 136, 150
  forms 42
calcium citrate malate 42
calcium glycinate 42
calcium-magnesium ratio 42, 43, 133
cancer 26, 27, 53, 54, 55, 57, 58, 59, 60, 61, 62, 63, 64, 65, 70, 71, 73, 81, 85, 86–87, 101, 103-120, 123, 125, 127, 133, 136, 144, 145
  mortality 15, 26, 105, 114–116, 118
  prevention 105–106
Candida 124, 128
canola oil 147
cardiomyopathy 28, 29
carnitine 95
catalytic hydrogenation 16, 141, 142, 143, 145
CD4 levels 80, 83, 85, 86, 88, 89, 90, 91, 92, 93, 94, 95, 96
CD8 *see* T-cells
cerevastatin 27
cheese 22, 133, 136–137
chelates 45
chemotherapy 103–120
  drug companies 112–113, 118
  evaluation 106–107, 108, 109, 119–120
  financial incentives 110-112
  side effects 104, 115, 116–117
  survival rates 104, 106-107, 108, 114–116, 119
  trials 107, 108–110, 115
cholecalciferol *see* vitamin D3
cholesterol 11, 14–15, 16, 17, 18, 19,

24–25, 26, 27, 30, 32, 44, 61, 81, 96, 128,136, 145, 147
  HDL ('good' cholesterol) 24, 29, 61, 146
  high blood levels 11, 15, 23, 24, 28–29, 30–31, 37, 141
  hormone production 30–31
  LDL ('bad' cholesterol) 15, 24–25, 35, 37, 61, 128, 146
  lowering 12, 14, 15, 16, 18, 19, 20, 23, 24, 25, 26, 28-29, 35, 128, 141
    drugs 18, 23, 24, 25, 26, 27, 29, 30
    see also statin drugs
  LPA 15, 24, 28, 32, 33, 35, 36, 37, 145
chromium 133
cisplatin 107, 115, 116
coconut
  milk 147
  oil 16
cod liver oil see fish oil
collagen 14, 31, 32, 33, 37, 41, 46
condom use 84, 97
conjugated horse estrogens 54, 55, 56–57, 59, 61, 62, 63, 64, 66 see also estrogens, Premarin
copper 43, 46, 71, 76, 150
coronary artery disease 11–37, 47, 55, 58, 70, 73, 133, 135, 145
  causes 11, 15, 16, 19, 141
    cholesterol 11, 15, 16, 17, 23–25, 141, 147
    fat theory 15–16, 18, 23
    hormone imbalance 30–31, 36

refined flour 13–14, 16
  smoking 13
facts about 14–15
incidence 11–12, 14, 16, 17, 18, 21, 22, 135, 146
mortality 11, 12, 14, 15, 16, 17, 19–20, 26, 35, 37, 105, 135
treatment 12, 26, 35
  vitamin C 33–34, 35
  trials 19, 20, 21, 26, 34, 142
coronary bypass operations 33–34
corticoid drugs 40, 49, 124
see also cortisone
cortisol 97
cortisone 49, 96, 124, 125
see also steroid hormones
Coxsackie virus 92, 100
Crohn's disease 127, 129
cysteine 88, 89, 90, 91, 93, 94
cytokines 71, 73, 127

DDC see antiretrovirals
DHEA (dihydroepiandrosterone) 24–25, 31, 71, 88, 96, 97
diabetes 13, 19, 20, 28 see also insulin
  childhood 133–34
diarrhoea 74, 93, 95, 123, 125, 126, 128, 129, 138
DNA 79–80, 93, 99, 136
doxorubicin 117

elastin 14, 31, 46

ERT *see* estrogen replacement therapy

essential fatty acids *see* omega fatty acids

estradiol 56, 57, 58, 61, 62, 63, 64, 65

estriol 50, 57, 58, 61, 62, 64, 65, 66

estrogen replacement therapy 53, 54, 57, 62–63, 64, 66

estrogens 24, 31, 39, 40, 46, 47, 49, 50, 53, 54, 55, 56-57, 58–59, 60, 63, 64, 65, 66, 71, 96, 132, 136

estrone 54, 56, 57, 58, 61, 62, 63, 64, 65

evening primrose oil 18, 135, 147

exercise 21, 29, 35, 40, 49

fatty acids *see* omega fatty acids

fibrinogen 32, 35, 36–37

fish oil 18, 37, 64, 71, 147

flavonoids *see* bioflavonoids

flaxseed oil 18, 147

fluoride 43, 46

folic acid 36, 47, 48, 50, 65, 71, 76, 117, 150

food industry 18–19, 106, 142, 145

free radicals 13, 15, 17, 75, 83, 89, 91, 95

GLA (gammacarboxyglutamic acid) 45

glucose 13, 28

glucuronic acid 54, 56

glutamine 88, 93, 94

glutathione (GSH) 89–90, 91, 92, 93, 94, 95

glutathione peroxidase 91, 92, 93, 100

glutathione reductase 91

glycaemic index 13

glycine 42, 89

glycol 37

glycoproteins 37, 41

heart attacks 11, 15, 18, 20, 21, 22, 23,24, 26, 28, 31, 33, 34-35, 36, 37, 44, 54, 59, 61, 64, 66, 71, 142, 143, 145, 146

helper T-cells *see* T-cells

haematocrit test 69, 70–71, 72–73

haemoglobin 70, 71, 73, 74

high-density lipoprotein *see* cholesterol – HDL

HIV 79–101 *see also* viruses

 diagnosis 82

 drug resistance 97

 facts about 79–80, 83–85

 incidence 79, 81, 84, 85

 infection rates 81, 83

 mother-to-child transmission 83, 86

 mutations 97, 98

 nutrient deficiencies 83, 88, 99–100

 prevention 79

 origins 83, 87–88

 treatment 79, 80, 81, 82, 97

vaccines 79, 80, 98–99

homocysteine 15, 32, 34, 35, 36, 37, 47, 48

hormone imbalances 24, 30–31, 36, 40, 71, 96

hormone replacement therapy 31, 49, 53–66

   alternatives 65–66

   safety 53, 56

   trials 53, 54, 55, 57

hormones *see* steroid hormones

horse estrogens *see* conjugated horse estrogens, Premarin

horse urine 54, 56

HRT *see* hormone replacement therapy

human immunodeficiency virus *see* HIV

hydroperoxides 17

hypercholesterolaemia *see* cholesterol – high blood levels

I

immune system 17, 28, 74, 80, 81, 84, 85, 86, 88, 90, 93, 96, 97, 104, 117, 119, 123, 124, 125-126, 133, 136

immunoglobins 125

indole-3-carbinol (I3C) 65

insulin 13, 28, 133

iron 15, 69, 71, 74, 75, 76

   infants 74–75, 124

K

Kaposi's sarcoma 86–87, 92

L

L-carnitine *see* carnitine

L-lysine *see* lysine

L-proline *see* proline

lactase 138

lactobacillus 124, 126, 128, 129, 134

lactose 138

lard 16, 18–19 *see also* saturated fats

lipoic acid 90, 95

low-density lipoprotein *see* cholesterol – LDL

lymphocytes 85, 90, 92, 93, 95, 125–126, 127

lysine 33, 34, 35

M

macrophages 125, 126, 127

magnesium 39, 41, 42, 43, 44, 46, 49, 85, 91, 131, 133, 149, 150

maize oil 16

manganese 43, 46, 133, 150

margarine 16, 17, 18–19, 20, 21, 22, 23, 141–147 *see also* polyunsaturated fats

   animal experiments 145

   cholesterol-lowering effect 16, 23, 141

   production 142–143

meat

   in diet 22, 49, 144

melatonin 71, 97

menopause 40, 43, 46, 53–54, 57, 58, 59, 64, 65, 66

mercury 85

methionine 36

methyl groups 36

mevalonate 27

micro-organisms *see* bacteria

milk 39, 40, 41, 42, 131–138 *see also*
breast milk
  fat 133, 136, 147
  homogenisation 132, 135, 136
  modern components 131–133, 136
  pasteurisation 132, 135

mitochondria 27, 95

molybdenum 136

monounsaturated fats 142

mucopolysaccharides 46

N-acetylcysteine (NAC) 37, 90,
91, 94

nutrient sources 149-150

olive oil 142, 147

omega fatty acids 13, 18, 134–135, 144
  dietary supplements 18, 64, 65,
71, 147

osteoblasts 46, 47

osteocalcin 41, 45

osteoclasts 47, 49

osteonectin 41

osteoporosis 39-50, 59–60, 64, 133
  incidence 13, 41
  prevention 39, 41, 42, 43, 46,

47, 48, 58, 66, 131, 138
supplement regime 49–50
treatment 39, 43, 44, 46, 47,
48, 150

peanut oil 22, 147

peripheral neuropathy 28

pesticides 132, 136, 144

pharmaceutical industry 18–19, 59, 82,
98, 109, 112–113, 118

phosphorus 43, 46

phytoestrogens *see* plant estrogens

plant estrogens 64–66 *see also*
Triple Estrogen

plaque 11, 14, 17, 23, 26,
32-33, 44
  artery walls 11, 14, 17, 32, 33,
131, 136
  vein walls 14, 32

Policosanol 29

polyunsaturated fats 16, 17, 18–19, 20,
21, 22, 23, 141, 142, 143, 146

pregnenolone 30, 31

Premarin 40, 47, 54, 55, 56–57, 58, 59,
61–63, 66

Prempro 53, 54, 55, 57

probiotics 123-129, 134, 136 *see also*
bifidobacteria, lactobacillus
  dosages 129

progesterone 31, 40, 47, 50, 54, 56,
60, 66

progestin 53, 54, 57, 60

progestogens 40, 47, 54, 55, 57, 59,
  60–61, 63, 66
proline 33, 35
prostaglandins 135, 144
protease inhibitors 97
Provera 57
Prudent Diet 18–20, 21, 22
    trials 19–20, 21
PUFAs *see* polyunsaturated fats

Q10 (coenzyme) 24, 27, 28, 30, 96
quercitin 17

refined carbohydrates 13, 15, 16, 23, 29,
  34, 35, 37, 49, 124, 125, 128, 135
reverse transcriptase 93, 95, 97
rhabdomyolosis 27
riboflavin 91
RNA 79–80, 93

S-adenosyl–methionine 90
saturated fats 16, 18, 19, 22, 23, 141,
  142, 145, 146
selenium 65, 85, 86, 87, 88, 90,
  91, 92, 93, 94, 99–101, 133
sesame oil 147
silicon 43, 46, 49
smoking 40, 49, 106

soy isoflavones 50, 65
soya milk 138
soya oil 143
statin drugs 23, 24, 25, 26, 29,
  30, 31
    alternatives 29–30
    side effects 27–28
steroid hormones 11, 30–31, 63, 97, 124
see also cortisone
strokes 24, 25, 29, 47, 54, 55, 64, 70,
  74, 143
sunflower oil 16, 142, 147
synergism 42, 64, 76
    nutrients 42–43, 89, 150

T-cells 28, 80, 85, 89, 99, 125, 126
see also CD4
T-lymphocytes see lymphocytes
testosterone 24, 31, 46, 49, 71, 96
tocopherols see vitamin E
trans fatty acids 143–144, 145, 146
triglycerides (TG) 29, 36, 37, 61, 62, 145
trimethyl glycine (betaine) 36
Triple Estrogen (Tri-E, Tri-Est) 64, 65, 66
tryptophan 88, 93, 95

viruses 79, 89, 91, 126
    replication 79–80, 83, 88, 92,
      93, 95
vitamin A 37, 64

vitamin B1 117, 150
vitamin B2 117, 150
vitamin B3 (niacin) 29, 91, 117, 150
vitamin B6 36, 47, 50, 71, 150
vitamin B12 36, 47, 50, 71, 76, 150
vitamin C 14, 24, 31-33, 37, 46–47,
  50, 63, 71, 90, 91, 97, 111, 115,
  116–117, 118, 119, 120
    and coronary artery disease 14, 24,
      31–33, 34, 35
    trials 34, 118
vitamin D *see* vitamin D3
vitamin D3 44, 45–46, 50, 64, 132, 135
vitamin E 13, 14, 16, 18, 24–25, 63, 64,
  71, 117
vitamin K 44–45, 46, 50, 71, 117
    sources 45

warfarin 45, 49
whey protein 90
wine
    and coronary artery disease 17

xanthine oxidase 136

zinc 41, 43, 46, 49, 71, 76, 150